THIS IS WHY YOU'RE
SICK & TIRED

ALSO BY JACKIE WARNER

This Is Why You're Fat *(And How to Get Thin Forever):*
Eat More, Cheat More, Lose More—and Keep the Weight Off

10 Pounds in 10 Days:
The Secret Celebrity Program for Losing Weight Fast

THIS IS WHY YOU'RE
SICK & TIRED

(AND HOW TO LOOK AND FEEL AMAZING)

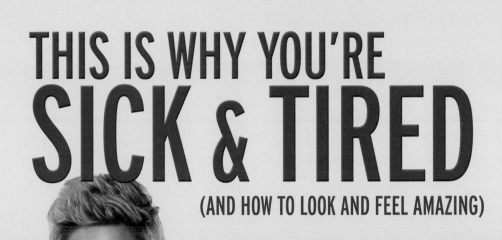

JACKIE WARNER

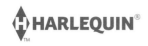

This Is Why You're Sick & Tired
(And How to Look and Feel Amazing)

ISBN-13: 978-0-373-89316-4

Cover photo and photos on pages xii, 70 and 137 by Blake Little
All other interior photos by Daveed Benito
Jackie Warner wardrobe by Elisabetta Rogiani

The health advice presented in this book is intended only as an informative resource guide to help you make informed decisions; it is not meant to replace the advice of a physician or to serve as a guide to self-treatment. Always seek competent medical help for any health condition or if there is any question about the appropriateness of a procedure or health recommendation.

Library of Congress Cataloging-in-Publication Data
Warner, Jackie, 1968-
  This is why you're sick & tired : (and how to look and feel amazing) / Jackie Warner.
     pages cm
  Includes bibliographical references and index.
  ISBN 978-0-373-89316-4 (hardback)
 1. Detoxification (Health) 2. Physical fitness. 3. Self-care, Health. I. Title.
  RA784.5.W37 2015
  613.2--dc23
                          2014030260

www.Harlequin.com

Printed in U.S.A.

CONTENTS

"WE HAVE BECOME FRUSTRATED, FRAZZLED AND UNHEALTHY"

INTRODUCTION

I've trained thousands of clients, worked with some of the biggest celebrities and operated top medical clinics for more than two decades. I have been in the trenches of weight loss and well-being, turning breakdowns to "breakthroughs." Everything I've learned has led me to write this book, which is a groundbreaking program to help *you* recapture your good health and energy.

You will learn the simple reasons that you are feeling less than great and the simple solutions to regaining vitality. I have been blessed to work in a preventive care industry where I get to help people "wake up" to a new truth and a new way of being. The life-changing program you'll find in this book includes all the tools in my arsenal to first give you an understanding of yourself and your body—and then give you a permanent solution for health and happiness.

IS THIS YOU?

My grandmother is from the South and has many colorful phrases for how people should live their lives. When she is really fed up with something and her frustration hits an intolerable level, she says, "Honey, I'm just sick and tired!" This sentiment is what I am hearing all over America—men and women are fed up with being literally sick and tired. We have become frustrated, frazzled and unhealthy—run-down and lacking the energy to live up to our true potential. Many of us feel like we are rats on wheels, striving to keep our heads above water while desperately trying to succeed at the things that matter most to us. For some, it's our careers; for others, it's our families, or the desire to partner and create a family. For many of us, it's both.

You may feel as if you are fighting an uphill battle with yourself, relying on quick fixes like energy drinks, processed foods and prescriptions to get you through your days. We are living in a highly stressful and chemical-infused country, where big companies make decisions based on the bottom line instead of our well-being. Technology has changed our society into a fast-moving freeway of constant information, with the average person checking his smartphone 150 times a day! This connection to the world is wonderful but has some serious side effects. The constant bombardment of information and communication through advertising and social media can have an anxiety-causing effect that makes your other lifestyle choices that much more important. It's a double-edged sword; our continual exposure to information, news (much of it bad) and chatter makes us anxious—but then being unable to "connect" makes us anxious, too! Take the recent research that found that 45 percent of people unable to access their social media networks or email felt worried, uncomfortable and anxious as a result.

We live in a "must-have-now society." The problem is that our biology has not fully adapted, and cellular breakdown, adrenal fatigue and sleep dysfunction are wearing us down. The creation of many foods, products and environments that cater to a busy lifestyle have startling and devastating effects on our biochemistry and emotions. The foods we automatically reach for and those that are easiest to find are all too often toxic to our bodies. This rampant exhaustion doesn't just ruin the quality of our lives today; it is also the warning sign and beginning of inflammation and chronic illness down the line. It's time to break free from the environmental and biological drains that keep us exhausted.

Being sick and tired makes us:

- ✖ Too tired to work out
- ✖ Too cloudy to make the best food decisions
- ✖ Too stressed to be happy and peaceful
- ✖ Too imbalanced to sleep deeply

Through the years, it's become very clear that our health crisis runs deeper than weight, to the very foundations of our energy and well-being. My clients don't come to me just so they can *look* amazing. They come to me so they can *feel* amazing. And the two go hand in hand.

I'll bet that you have spent a lot of time and energy attempting to start a better lifestyle but low energy absolutely affects your ability to set and reach your goals. You will learn that a lot of things you *thought* were right are actually wrong, causing your body to function at constant "red alert." In this program you will learn how to:

+ Reinvigorate cells and glands
+ Have a body that's lean and clean
+ Sleep like a baby

BEAUTIFUL FROM THE INSIDE OUT

In *This Is Why You're Sick & Tired*, I have created a super-detox, three-phase plan to kick off your new, healthy lifestyle. You'll find fun and easy recipes that will instantly give you more energy. The 21-Day Detox is carefully designed to restore and recharge your body so you look and feel amazing. You will learn exactly how and what to eat in order to reboot a sluggish system and operate at your peak capacity. Feeling up and alert during the day and sleeping well at night will leave you feeling more positive and happier. And, oh yeah, you will drop that extra weight fast and look amazing.

In a very short time, balance and brightness can be reclaimed. When physical and psychological reserves are rebuilt, life feels brand-new. I've seen it in thousands of people—the transformation that takes place when they've gone from "burn out" to "burn bright." And I'm talking about a brightness that doesn't fade—a constant state of vitality that allows people to perform and recover in circumstances that would have crushed them before. Family challenges, work stress, illness, weight management—you'll be able to handle all of them skillfully and with a new sense of strength and confidence.

A PROGRAM THAT'S BETTER THAN MEDICINE

Let me share with you how the journey I took in writing this book started. My mother told me something her doctor had said to her during a regular exam: "When people come to us with 'lifestyle diseases,' we prescribe medication to treat them. Then, when the side effects make them sicker, we prescribe more medication to treat the side effects."

I already knew that many drugs throw off our bodies' systems and cause deeper health issues. What made me sad was how powerless our doctors feel when it comes to preventive care. The truth is that most of our doctors aren't educated enough on how to prevent disease—they just treat it. Many doctors have complained to me that they feel insufficiently trained in nutrition and that they feel forced to treat symptoms with meds once a person is already sick or diseased. A healthy lifestyle is just not the focus of medical school, but it should be.

All too often, the pills that people take to feel better end up pushing them further into the sick and tired spiral. Mood stabilizers can have the most serious effects on well-being, creating constant fatigue, lack of motivation and a pervasive sense of numbness. The problem is that these pills are usually prescribed before lifestyle remedies are even suggested—despite all evidence that diet and exercise can completely, positively transform how people view themselves and their lives.

THE SOLUTION

The solution doesn't come in a bottle. It comes from my thoroughly researched, specific three-phase eating plan that shows you clearly how to eat for a total transformation. Each week will offer a new diet and exercise program that alters your biochemistry in stages, working with your brain and body to balance and release a new set of chemicals and patterns. The diet has been carefully coupled with a progressive style of training that adapts and changes each week, along with your foods and your body chemistry. Once you have completed the reset, you will be fully prepared to live a whole new lifestyle—one that is energetic and positive!

Here's the 21-Day Detox program at a glance:

+ In Phase 1: **Detox & Prime**, the focus is on cellular rehab and rejuvenation. This all-vegan detox diet is abundant in foods that are easily broken down during digestion, to maximize nutrient absorption and create supercharged cells. The workouts are based on light power circuit training, designed to prime internal systems for the next stage of intensity.

+ In Phase 2: **Balance & Burn**, metabolism- and mood-related hormones are recalibrated and your body clock is retuned, increasing calm, boosting energy and bettering sleep. The eating plan this week focuses on normalizing out-of-whack adrenal and thyroid functions, and on regulating insulin response. Workouts are based on multijoint movements, engaging the maximum amount of muscle fibers, incinerating fat, increasing overall weight loss and deepening sleep.

+ In Phase 3: **Lean & Mean**, you'll experience the ultimate in muscle shaping and strengthening. Each meal is designed to prompt a different chemical reaction at different times of the day to work with your body's natural circadian rhythms. For example, breakfast and lunch contain energy-sustaining foods, while dinners and evening snacks contain foods that trigger dopamine and serotonin, the body's natural relaxants. Your workouts include my specially designed Power Ladders, a method of training that takes you to muscle failure, creating rapid increases in muscle building and tone.

My powerful program will transform you from the dysfunctional, dissatisfied person you have become to the energetic, strong and sexy person you were meant to be. So, if you're buying this book to get a great body, you've made a good investment. If you're buying this book because you just feel crappy and don't know how to change, then you are on your way to a significant awakening. It's time for you to gain the knowledge of how to take control of your body and your life once and for all. With this new knowledge, it is totally possible to manifest a different destiny for yourself.

This Is Why You're Sick & Tired will give you the key to unlock a new, improved you!

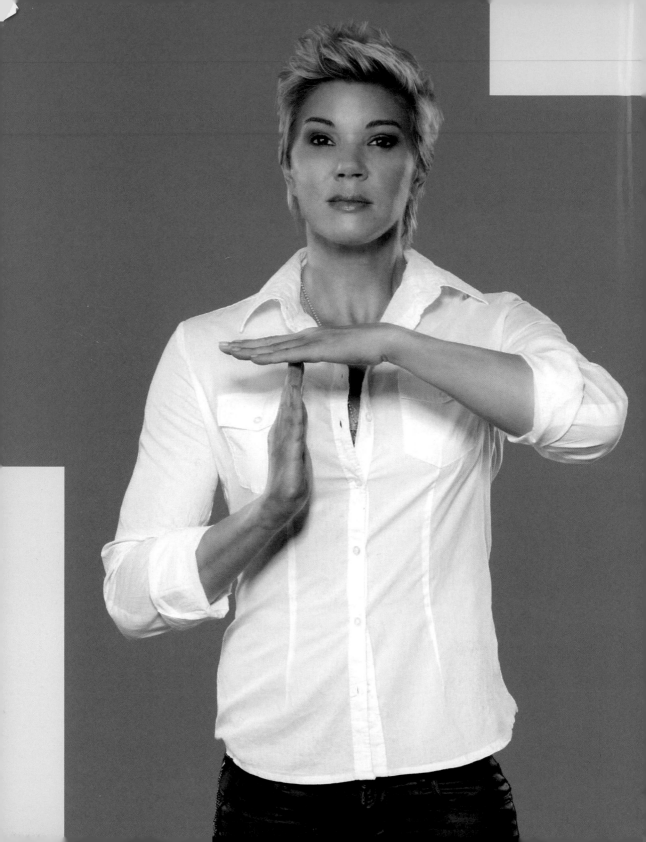

PART ONE

WHY YOU'RE SICK & TIRED

" YOUR CELLS ARE RESPONSIBLE FOR EVERY FUNCTION **INVOLVING ENERGY, WEIGHT AND METABOLISM** "

CHAPTER ONE

WHEN GOOD CELLS GO BAD

Do you feel sick, depressed, run-down or anxious? Well, so do your cells! They are experiencing the same problems at the cellular level— and causing most of your external symptoms.

The fact is that human beings were not intended to survive past middle age. From our Paleolithic ancestors until about a hundred years ago, the average life span ranged between 20 and 40 years old. Life span began to rise in the 19th century, hitting 49 in the United States in 1900, and then it took off in the 20th century. This is largely due to breakthroughs in medicine.

Today, the average baby born in this country will live to 78. The average 35-year-old will live to about 80. And the average 65-year-old will live past 83. Medical breakthroughs and discoveries have enabled us to live longer lives than ever before. The problem is that our cells haven't been able to "catch up" to these new life spans. Each passing year our cells degrade and that degradation accelerates after the age of 40! Without a healthy lifestyle intervention, our quality of life is severely compromised.

Your cells are responsible for every function involving energy, weight and metabolism. When they're broken, all the systems that depend on them break, too. Bad cells stall energy, undermine weight management and cause early aging. The problem is that modern society drastically degrades cell health. Consider the following assaults on our cell health:

- ✖ Stress
- ✖ Processed foods
- ✖ Environmental toxins
- ✖ Antibiotics
- ✖ Excess coffee, alcohol and sugar consumption

All corrupt cell integrity. Simply put, your cells will still work to keep you alive, but if they're broken down, your quality of life will be severely compromised.

When cells are fed up, they go on strike and stop cleansing the body of the built-up "trash." Systems supporting immunity, energy, youth and mood will function only at about 30 percent, instead of 100 percent. Here are the two main issues causing toxic cells that we will be healing:

1 Your cells have been denied vital nutrients, and are starving to death.

2 Your cells have been poisoned, and are malfunctioning, wreaking havoc on your brain and body.

To understand what's happening in your cells, let's take a closer look inside them. There are more than 200 different types of cells in your body, which differ in size, shape and function. Human cells handle stress the same way people handle stress. Just like people, they can survive under horrible circumstances but rarely can they thrive under those circumstances. *You* need to give them extra TLC to counter this modern, toxic society.

Your very quality of life may depend on the quality of your cells. Cells crave proper nutrients, water and oxygen. If they are fed and oxygenated appropriately, they will expunge waste efficiently and they will communicate beautifully with one another. This means that your brain and body will start functioning like they were born to—perfectly in balance.

The cell is very complex and is made up of several parts called organelles. This program will enhance the entire cell, but I have chosen to focus on three key components that, when functioning well, will give you optimal energy and health.

THE BIG 3

+ Mitochondria (energy)

+ Nucleus (disease/DNA)

+ Cellular membrane (mood)

In an unhealthy cell, the functioning of these organelles decreases in an alarming way. The cellular garbage piles up and your body becomes toxic. Your immunity weakens and you consistently look and feel crappy. The cell can't produce sufficient ATP (energy) so you don't have the energy to consistently work out, care for your family the way you want to or aggressively pursue your dreams. The cell can't sufficiently synthesize protein, carbs and fat the way it's designed to; this means that you will gain weight and be unable to lose it. And then there is what I feel is the worst outcome of a degenerated cell: it cannot communicate appropriate chemical messages, leading to mood issues such as anxiety and depression.

EXHAUSTED

 LOW BATTERIES = **Run-down**

The mitochondria are the cellular power plants that use energy from the food you eat to produce energy called adenosine triphosphate, or ATP. ATP is the energy transport system within the body. In a healthy body, ATP is a fast-moving and efficient subway line carrying energy to all cells throughout the body. When mitochondria are not at full power, ATP transport is slow and low. This means *you* are slow and low! ATP controls metabolism, the very functioning of the body, from breathing to nutrient storage to chemical reactions. So the connection is this:

 LOW MITOCHONDRIA = Low ATP = Sluggish Metabolism = Run-down/Overweight

Mitochondria help you manage two types of fatigue—lack of stamina for performing daily tasks and delayed postexertional fatigue, which happens after you have expended a high dose of energy for a certain period. This could happen after a long day with the kids, a day at a high-stress job or an intense workout. If the mitochondria are not producing enough ATP, you will feel constantly run-down and exhausted. Dieting becomes an uphill battle that you never seem to win.

Depending on your mitochondria's "battery charge," you'll either be dragging all day long or have the energy and clarity to take on the world. Let's look at two factors that affect mitochondria.

TOO MANY FREE RADICALS

We will discuss free radicals in relation to sickness and disease later on, but now let's focus on their effect on energy. A healthy number of free radicals aid in fighting disease and cellular destruction, and provide energy. Unfortunately, our current lifestyle choices have caused an overproduction of free radicals. Think of too many free radicals as a rebel army that has gained too much power and is overthrowing its own government. (The mitochondrial creation of energy also creates some free radicals in the process, but these are easily combated by healthy cells.)

We're exposed to many things today that cause free radical damage, including:

- Fried foods
- A high-fat diet
- Consistent or excessive sugar intake
- Sun exposure
- Motor vehicle exhaust
- Smoking
- Drinking alcohol
- Stress
- Lack of sleep

When free radicals attack the mitochondria and DNA is damaged and mutated, your mitochondria's ability to produce energy is compromised. When mitochondria lose their ability to produce energy, you lose your energy as well. What happens on the microlevel expresses itself in your daily life. You become fatigued and run-down.

TOO LITTLE OXYGEN

A healthy cell is an oxygenated cell. Just as you need oxygen to live, so do your body's cells. Without oxygen, your mitochondria can't produce the energy that powers your cells—and powers you! Imagine someone with an asthma attack—he's unable to get the oxygen his body needs, so he can't function. The same thing happens with your body's cells. Normally, we get enough oxygen to power our body's cells through the air we breathe; it's then transported to our body's cells. But there are plenty of conditions that cut the amount of this vital molecule.

Factors that cause low oxygen in mitochondria are:

- ✖ Obesity
- ✖ Lack of exercise
- ✖ Sleep apnea
- ✖ Smoking
- ✖ Asthma and respiratory allergies
- ✖ Anemia

The cell detox diet will include mitochondria boosters, such as:

- ✚ Vitamin B_6
- ✚ Vitamin B_{12}
- ✚ Coenzyme Q10 (CoQ10)
- ✚ Zinc
- ✚ Folic acid

The goal is to wake up with high energy and maintain that level throughout the day, no matter what your exertion output is. When your mitochondria are producing high levels of ATP (energy), then you are actually being fueled by the things that used to wear you out. Your job becomes challenging in a good way and you feel energized by the high you get from doing it well. You leave the gym feeling amazing and happy you worked out. If you're a parent, you will have happier, lighter moments with your family. Mighty mitochondria mean that you are no longer in survival mode, but instead are the captain of your own ship!

SICK

NUCLEAR NUCLEUS

If you think of the mitochondria of the cell as its battery, then the nucleus of the cell is like the brain. It contains DNA, the blueprint and instructions of life. I wrote extensively about DNA expression in my last book, *10 Pounds in 10 Days,*

> **" TOXINS SUCH AS PESTICIDES AND OTHER CHEMICALS CAN CROSS THE CELLULAR MEMBRANE AND DAMAGE THE DNA, CAUSING IT TO BREAK OR FRAGMENT "**

because it is astonishing to me that researchers now know that what we eat— the foods we choose and how much we consume—can affect and transform our genes and cause disease and weight gain. For instance, we now know exactly what foods help turn off genes responsible for triggering inflammation in the body. In the meantime, we know that a diet high in fruits and vegetables, healthy fats and whole grains will keep our genes as healthy as possible. We now know that specific foods can change certain genes that we were born with and alter destructive genes that cause disease and weight gain.

The nucleus, which is surrounded by its own membrane, contains all the information your cell needs to thrive, and your cell cannot function without it. It is the brain of the cell. Different cells have different functions, and the DNA basically gives the cell its orders.

However, as you'll see, when we talk about the cellular membrane, we see that DNA is subject to attack. Toxins such as pesticides and other chemicals can cross the cellular membrane and damage the DNA, causing it to break or fragment. Free radicals, or reactive oxygen species (ROS), can cause the same kind of damage, called mutation. Mutated DNA messes up the "orders" your cell receives, and causes the cell to malfunction and even become cancerous. This leads to autoimmune disorders, diseases and even death.

AUTOIMMUNE EPIDEMIC

Nuclear DNA is susceptible to attack from free radicals, such as those produced by pollution, pesticides, food chemical additives, plastics and other toxins. When the nuclear DNA gets attacked, bad things happen, including the development of autoimmune disorders.

It seems that every time you turn on the TV, you see a new drug for the treatment of one autoimmune disorder or another. In fact, I worked with the National Psoriasis Foundation to create a healthy diet and exercise program for psoriasis sufferers. I couldn't believe how many young and seemingly healthy people were getting this horrible disorder!

Part of the reason for psoriasis and other autoimmune disorders may be that the nuclear DNA's blueprint has been compromised. If this DNA isn't functioning properly, your cells can't function properly, either. Take your T cells, which are an essential part of your immune system—they make sure that your immune system is reacting appropriately to toxins and other invaders. When T cells malfunction, though, they cause your immune system to overreact and even attack your own normal, healthy cells—and that leads to what we call "autoimmune disease."

Today there are an estimated 50–60 million Americans with autoimmune disorders, a huge increase from the estimated 8.5 million people who had autoimmune disorders in the mid-1990s. Here are some common autoimmune disorders:

✖ **Fibromyalgia.** This disorder strikes about 6 million Americans, most of them women. People with fibromyalgia suffer from constant pain throughout their body, fatigue and trouble sleeping. They also have memory problems and may suffer from depression, anxiety and irritable bowel syndrome.

* **Lupus.** About 1.5 million Americans have lupus, which occurs when your immune system goes haywire and attacks your healthy tissue. In most cases, doctors can't determine what causes the condition, but its symptoms include fatigue, fever, joint pain, skin lesions that worsen with sun exposure, chest pain, headaches, confusion, memory loss, dry eyes, shortness of breath, and fingers and toes that over-react to cold.

* **Chronic fatigue syndrome (CFS).** It is estimated that over a million Americans have chronic fatigue syndrome, which has similar symptoms to lupus. People with CFS suffer from fatigue, memory loss, trouble concentrating, sore throat, unexplained muscle and joint pain, bad headaches and unrefreshing sleep.

* **Psoriasis.** There are different types of psoriasis, but they all involve red, patchy, scaly skin or dry, cracked skin; burning, soreness or itching; and swollen or stiff joints. About 8.5 million Americans have psoriasis, which tends to go in cycles, called "flares."

* **Thyroid conditions.** Autoimmune disorders such as Graves' disease and Hashimoto's disease cause thyroid problems. Hyperthyroidism, a condition in which your body's thyroid gland produces too much thyroid hormone, and hypothyroidism, when it makes too little of that hormone, affect about 20 million Americans.

If you have an autoimmune disorder, you may be struggling just to *manage* your symptoms, and think that you have a lifelong sentence of doom. *But many of the symptoms you experience can be controlled—even eliminated—by the diet in this program.* You don't have to suffer. You just have to change your lifestyle and you'll see a huge difference in how you feel, both physically and emotionally!

DISEASED NATION

Degraded DNA may also lead to frightening diseases such as cancer, heart disease, liver disease, diabetes and Alzheimer's. Alzheimer's alone has increased tenfold throughout the last century, and is supposed to continue to increase 40 percent in the coming years. We are shocked to see that people who seemingly look healthy (like Tom Hanks) are being diagnosed with debilitating disease such as diabetes.

If mitochondria become damaged or swollen (a type of reversible cell damage), they not only leave you running on empty, but they also produce more free radicals. As I mentioned previously, these free radicals attack the cell's nucleus. Science shows that almost all degenerative diseases have their origin in dysfunctional free radical reactions.

Free radicals are everywhere—in the air, our bodies and the materials around us. They cause the deterioration of everything from plastics and wood to our bodies. It's more the external sources of free radicals—processed foods, exposure to chemicals and radiation, smoking and stress—that produce the free radicals that attack the nucleus of each of our cells. Chemicals, especially those that are fat-soluble, can also pass through the cellular membranes, including the nuclear membrane, and mutate your DNA.

Our mutated, degraded DNA is destroying our health. Take a look at your possible future if you don't stop the ravages of free radicals. Here's your lifetime risk of developing one of these often-fatal diseases:

CANCER—44 percent risk for men and 38 percent risk for women

HEART DISEASE—50 percent risk for men and 30 percent risk for women

ALZHEIMER'S—9 percent risk for men and 17 percent risk for women

DIABETES—33 percent risk for men and 40 percent risk for women

AUTOIMMUNE DISORDERS—5 percent risk for men and 8 percent risk for women

DAMAGED CELLS = Damaged Children

Scarier still, damaged DNA can be passed on when you have children. We now have a startling number of children with autism-related conditions—1 in 110—and 20 percent of children are diagnosed with a mental disorder. My research on this topic is very personal to me, as I am going through my third round of fertility treatments.

I am particularly interested in how to pass on good genetics and decrease risk to my baby. When I started this process, I was shocked at how many children are born with mutations and developmental problems. My findings all support what I already knew—lifestyle has a tremendous impact on cellular DNA. Here are some of my findings:

1 When DNA is damaged, essential reproductive functions (like the quality of your follicles, which become eggs in women and sperm in men) are negatively affected as well. This may be responsible for the increasing numbers of kids diagnosed with attention deficit/hyperactivity disorder (ADHD), which is as high as 7 percent!

2 Damaged DNA creates a higher risk for autism. People with autism tend to have a higher level of inflammation, a condition where your body is reacting to perceived immune threats. New research has found that at least some children (roughly one-third) with autism developed it while in the womb, when their immune systems were being developed, and this may be due to mutated DNA.

3 There's also a strong genetic component that influences whether your child will develop allergies or asthma. If you pass on damaged DNA, it ups the risk that your child will develop these conditions.

Simply put, how well we age and how healthy we are depend on the integrity of the cell. My cell detox diet will use very specific foods containing free radical scavengers such as:

+ B-complex vitamins
+ Ascorbic acid (vitamin C)
+ Alpha-tocopherol (vitamin E)
+ Beta-carotene

+ Coenzyme Q10
+ Enzymes, such as catalase and superoxide
+ Key minerals, such as selenium and zinc

COMMUNICATION BREAKDOWN

The cellular membrane is the skin of the cell. A healthy cell has a flexible, strong membrane that encloses each cell, protecting its internal elements so they can function properly. It allows nutrients to enter and wastes to be expelled. A healthy membrane is also essential for communication between your body's cells. Here's why.

Your membrane houses neurotransmitter transporters, which are like the smartphone hardware sending out text messages. Each cell sends and receives these chemical texts, which are directives on how and when to function.

If your membrane isn't healthy, though, those texts don't get through, or they wind up going to the wrong "phone." In your brain, that means that a message like "Hey, we need more serotonin," which regulates mood, sleep, sexuality and appetite, doesn't get delivered.

Much new research shows that depression and anxiety disorders stem from too much or too little of certain neurotransmitters (such as dopamine, norepinephrine and serotonin) in the brain, and researchers now believe that a stiff or torn cellular membrane interferes with their function, causing a host of symptoms. As you saw above, when we talked about the cell's nucleus, fat-soluble toxins that can permeate the membrane also interfere with communication.

AMERICANS ARE DEPRESSED!

More people are being diagnosed with depression than ever before. About 1 in 10 Americans will suffer from major depression every year, and 15–20 percent of both men and women experience depressive disorders, which are defined as depressed mood that lasts at least two years and includes conditions such as postpartum depression and seasonal affective disorder (SAD). The drug industry is making a killing trying to treat depression—22 million women alone are taking antidepressants.

" OVER 80 PERCENT OF THE PEOPLE WHO HAVE SYMPTOMS OF CLINICAL DEPRESSION ARE **NOT RECEIVING ANY SPECIFIC TREATMENT** "

Depression is more than a mental health problem. People with depression are more likely to have other serious health conditions, such as obesity, heart disease and stroke; they're also more likely to be unemployed or divorced than their peers.

DEPRESSION CAN LEAD TO ADDICTION

Despite the overmedication for depression, over 80 percent of the people who have symptoms of clinical depression are not receiving any specific treatment. Most people who are depressed do not take antidepressants. They self medicate, using other harmful coping mechanisms that give a spike of serotonin, such as fattening foods, alcohol and marijuana. This can lead to obesity and addiction. Eventually, these coping tools will cause your life to spiral out of control.

It's normal to want to feel better when you feel lousy, but self-medication only works in the short term. Sure, you feel better after a few drinks or a high-fat meal, but the next day you typically feel worse. Plus, many of the things we reach for when we're depressed actually worsen the symptoms we experience. Alcohol, for example, is actually a depressant. In the short term, you feel better, but after more than a couple of drinks, you're more depressed. Yet you're more likely to reach for that drink again because of the short-term relief of your symptoms. In fact, there is a very strong link between depression and drug and alcohol abuse.

Don't be one of these statistics! And if you already are, it's time to turn the ship around and heal your cells!

Signs of depression include:

- ✖ Ongoing feelings of sadness, anxiety or the "blahs"
- ✖ Feeling hopeless or pessimistic
- ✖ Loss of interest in hobbies and activities you used to enjoy
- ✖ Feeling guilty, worthless or helpless
- ✖ Difficulty concentrating or making decisions
- ✖ Memory problems
- ✖ Fatigue, decreased energy
- ✖ Insomnia, inability to stay asleep, desire to sleep all the time
- ✖ Changes in appetite and/or weight (either gaining or losing weight)
- ✖ Thoughts of death or suicide
- ✖ Suicide attempts
- ✖ Restlessness, irritability
- ✖ Headaches
- ✖ Muscle aches or unexplained achiness in body and joints
- ✖ Indigestion
- ✖ Shortness of breath

While the exact cause of depression is unknown, we know that it involves the balance of neurotransmitters such as dopamine, norepinephrine and serotonin. Anxiety and depression are often thought of as two sides of the same coin. When you are experiencing the above symptoms, you may become consistently anxious, which can lead to an anxiety disorder.

About one in five people each year suffers from symptoms related to anxiety disorders such as generalized anxiety disorder, obsessive-compulsive disorder and social anxiety disorder. While different disorders produce different symptoms, common signs of anxiety include:

- ✖ Difficulty relaxing and concentrating
- ✖ Constantly worrying about everyday problems
- ✖ Sleep problems
- ✖ Feeling "on edge," irritable, tense

* Fatigue
* Headaches
* Muscle tension or aches
* Nausea and/or indigestion
* Trembling
* Difficulty swallowing
* Shortness of breath

Unhealthy cellular membranes interfere with the normal communication process between the cells, which may be a cause of anxiety. Once again the messages that ask for more serotonin and other neurotransmitters don't get delivered, and the lack of those essential brain chemicals causes anxiety disorders. A healthy membrane helps maintain an even, balanced mood, despite the stresses of daily life.

Now that you know what is happening to your cells and the negative effects that has on your brain and body, let's look at the two-pronged cause. The two major factors of cell toxicity come from inside your body—from the foods you eat—and from outside your body—from the poisons and chemicals in your environment. When you understand how these internal and external factors destroy your cells, you'll want to change everything you can—within reason—to protect your body's essential functions!

FOOD POISONING

If you live and eat in America, you are probably starving and poisoning your cells. Our food industry is so corrupt and greedy that much of what we consume is full of disease-causing chemicals that keep our body in a toxic state and damage our DNA.

There are three types of foods destroying your cells:

* Processed foods
* Factory-farmed foods
* Pesticides

PROCESSED FOODS

These are foods that need to be processed extensively to be edible and are not found in nature. These foods aren't grown; they're manufactured. The food industry is not concerned about the impact these chemicals have on your health; they are only concerned about making a profit. In the 1950s and 1960s, food manufacturers needed to be able to feed a growing population and make more food faster and more cheaply. They found that by adding chemicals and other additives to food, it would stay "fresh" longer and retain its taste and flavor.

Now there are 10,000 artificial substances currently allowed in food! In fact, the FDA allows many additives that have been banned in other countries. If you're eating something packaged in plastic, chances are it contains additives, artificial flavorings and other chemical ingredients.

Processed foods are filled with unhealthy chemicals, but here are the three worst offenders:

✖ **Artificial dyes** such as Blue 1, Blue 2, Red 3 and Yellow 6. They make food more colorful (think kids' cereals and macaroni and cheese), but they're also linked to cancer and cell damage.

✖ **Potassium bromide.** This is added to flour to decrease baking time, but it's been linked to cancer, nervous system damage and kidney damage.

✖ **Butylated hydroxyanisole (BHA) and butylated hydroxytoluene (BHT).** These chemical preservatives are known carcinogens, or cancer-causers.

Basically, nearly anything that is boxed or portable, that is marketed as a quick and delicious meal or snack, is processed. In the last 25 years, chemical additives have flourished, and so has the rate of mental illness such as depression and anxiety.

Chemical additives are found in foods such as:

* Cookies and other baked goods
* Most cereals
* Most frozen meals
* Most canned goods
* Most boxed meals
* Most convenience meals and snacks

I realize that sometimes you need to grab something on the run, and that it's nearly impossible to completely avoid all processed foods. My program, though, will help rebuild your cells so that they're able to better defend themselves against the chemicals and additives you're exposed to.

FACTORY-FARMED FOODS

Out of all of the many ways the food industry is poisoning us, there is none as destructive to our cells as the current method of livestock and poultry raising: factory farming. I've always known about factory farming (a system of rearing livestock using restrictive methods, by which poultry, pigs or cattle are confined indoors under strictly controlled conditions), but as I conducted research for this book, I was so horrified by the level of cruelty to animals that I burst into tears.

I will not share with you the graphic and disgusting ways we treat our farm animals in America. If you want to learn more, simply do an online search for "factory farming." It will strengthen your desire to eat free-range meats or, if you don't have that option, no meat at all! My definition of a good person is someone who causes the least amount of suffering and pain possible in the world—and finds ways to lessen the pain and suffering in the world that is already present. I do not judge anyone who makes decisions without knowledge, but when you learn how cruel the factory farm industry is, I'm fairly certain you will change your eating habits! Lecture over. My job is to simply tell you what the end result of this animal mistreatment is on your body and how to drastically repair your health and increase your energy. Here are four ways our meat is being poisoned.

1. GRAIN-FED ANIMALS

I recently rescued a puppy and when I took him to the vet for a checkup, she cautioned me to *not* feed him dog food that has any grains or fillers. Apparently grain-fed dogs have a shorter life span and are more likely to die due to disease.

Now let's take that a step further and discuss what effect grains have on our livestock and poultry. Until very recently, our ancestors ate meat, poultry and fish. The animals they ate grazed on what they were supposed to—their natural food sources for each species. Today factory farms do everything they can to produce more meat from fewer animals, and that means interfering with the animals' natural diets and health. Factory farms feed animals not what they evolved to eat, but whatever food is the cheapest—and that's almost always grain.

Factory-farmed poultry and meat are fed grains to fatten them up more quickly, which abnormally alters the ratios of essential fatty acids. Livestock fed on grain have less omega-3 fat, which is beneficial for cardiac health, and more omega-6 fat, which may promote heart disease, in their tissues. When you eat grain-fed meat, you get even more omega-6 fats in your diet, which is not healthy.

2. HORMONES FOR WEIGHT GAIN

Various combinations of the natural hormones—estradiol, progesterone and testosterone—and the synthetic hormones—zeranol and trenbolone acetate—are given to cattle and poultry during their growing cycle. When humans eat this drug- and hormone-tainted beef or poultry, they consume these hormones. Human consumption of estrogen from hormone-drugged beef can result in estrogen dominance, a condition where you have too much estrogen in your body, compared to other hormones. Signs of estrogen dominance include weight gain, fatigue, memory problems, mood swings, bloating and headaches.

3. ANTIBIOTICS

It's not only hormones that are pumped into the animals we eat; they're full of antibiotics as well. The goal of factory farms is to produce as much meat as possible in as little space, for as little money. That means that animals are crowded together in pens where they are often unable to move.

Most of the breeding sows in the United States are confined in crates that are two feet by seven feet long. Dairy cattle are removed from their calves immediately and are milked two to three times a day; although normally they would live to about 25 years old, after four or five years they are killed for low-grade meat because their bodies have been "spent" producing so many calves. Egg-laying chickens are housed in "battery cages" that are so small their muscles atrophy from lack of use; they're unable to even turn around. And chickens raised for meat don't have it much better; they're crammed into windowless buildings by the thousands, where they spend their brief lives pecking each other and standing in their own excrement.

Are you sick to your stomach yet? It's not just how the animals are treated—the overcrowding and filthy conditions cause all kinds of infections, so the animals are pumped full of antibiotics. The largest use of antibiotics (over 50 percent of all antibiotic use!) in the United States is for animals. Routine antibiotic use is contributing to the growing problem of antibiotic resistance in humans.

Those antibiotics are then passed along to us when we eat factory-farmed meat, and this is dangerous for several reasons. First off, the antibiotics don't even work! A 2011 study found that nearly half of the meat and poultry in grocery stores contained S. aureus, or "staph," which causes staph infections in people. Second, the overuse of antibiotics causes resistant bacteria, or "superbacteria," which can't be killed with the drugs most often used to fight them. This makes you more likely to develop a bacterial condition that is difficult to treat, and possibly even fatal. Third, animals produce an enormous amount of waste, which contains antibiotics and superbugs that then get into the groundwater and environment and are again passed onto people unfortunate enough to live near factory farms.

4. IRRADIATION CAUSES CARCINOGENIC BY-PRODUCTS

Factory-farmed meat is treated with radioactive material (e.g., gamma rays) or electricity in order to kill bacteria brought on by squalid conditions. Exposing food to radioactive waves destroys not only bacteria, but splits molecules into smaller parts, creating carcinogenic, or cancer-causing, by-products. We know that there are health risks to x-rays and radiation. A pregnant woman cannot even have her mouth x-rayed for fear of harming the fetus. Cancer rates in the United States continue to rise, and irradiated food is likely playing a role in this increase.

Maybe this has put you off eating meat forever—or at least made you want to eat meat that is free of hormones and antibiotics. My program will show you how to get plenty of quality protein if you decide to go without meat, and teach you how to find meat and poultry that's organically and humanely raised. Your health will improve and you'll do something good for animals and the environment, too.

PESTICIDES

Pesticides are used to kill bugs, birds and animals that are attracted to produce. They affect the nervous system by disrupting key enzymes. They became widely used after World War II. The government saw what neurotoxins did to the enemy and allowed farmers to administer those same poisons to our produce as a pest deterrent. Are you starting to see a pattern here? When it comes to common sense and human welfare, the government is sadly lacking!

Pesticides are absorbed in fat cells and are not excreted, so you retain them for a lifetime. Studies show that pesticide exposure is strongly linked to the following:

* Cancer
* Neurological defects
* Fertility problems
* Birth defects
* Fetal death
* Neurodevelopmental disorders, such as autism, Down syndrome, communication disorders and attention deficit/hyperactivity disorder

The American Medical Association recommends limiting exposure to pesticides and using safer alternatives instead. According to the AMA, "Particular uncertainty exists regarding the long-term effects of low-dose pesticide exposures."

Pesticides clearly represent a huge threat to our health—and our children's—but I'll show you how to lessen your exposure to these toxins and to help your body's cells combat them when they are exposed! Remember, healthy cells can protect themselves from just about any pesticide or other poison.

Some fruits and veggies are more likely to be loaded with pesticides than others. Here are the top 14 most toxic fruits and veggies, dubbed the Dirty Dozen (Plus 2) by the Environmental Working Group:

- ✖ Apples
- ✖ Celery
- ✖ Cherry tomatoes
- ✖ Cucumbers
- ✖ Grapes
- ✖ Hot peppers
- ✖ Kale/collard greens
- ✖ Nectarines (imported)
- ✖ Peaches
- ✖ Potatoes
- ✖ Spinach
- ✖ Strawberries
- ✖ Sweet bell peppers
- ✖ Summer squash

Pesticide/ Autism Link

A 2007 study by the California Department of Public Health found that women in the first eight weeks of pregnancy who live near farm fields sprayed with pesticides were several times more likely to give birth to children with autism.

Just as if you were secretly and slowly being poisoned by arsenic, you are being poisoned by the food industry. These poisons give rise to similar symptoms: fatigue, low immunity and an emergency response by the body. Consuming these toxic foods causes the cells of the body to stop functioning properly, degrading energy metabolism and organ and tissue function.

But just as there is bad news, there is good news. My plan will show you how to avoid the worst of the worst, and choose the best of not-so-great options. Plus, you'll learn which foods will supercharge your cells' ability to fight back against the things that would normally poison them.

THE CHEMICAL SPILL (PACKAGE POISONS)

We've talked about the substances we ingest through the foods we eat, but there's another danger to our cells—the poisons, toxins and chemicals we're exposed to on a daily basis. A hundred years ago we didn't have to worry about pesticides, parabens and other chemicals. Today if you live in a developed country, you're exposed to human-made toxins created to kill living things, not to mention all the other human-made chemicals used in manufacturing that eventually wind up in our bodies.

Your cells are designed to defend against and adapt to extreme hazards, but when a dirty world and food supply overburden the body so much that its cleansing system stops working, the result is a total breakdown in energy and immunity.

People drink, eat and breathe hundreds of invisible environmental toxins daily. Our safety standards for consumable products and foods are well below what many third world countries allow. We are literally getting poisoned daily. Almost all lotions and hair and beauty products contain toxic parabens. I'm not asking you to stop using these beauty products because, quite frankly, it's nearly impossible. I am asking you to give up one thing—water bottles.

WATER BOTTLES

Most plastics, including water bottle plastics, contain Bisphenol A, or BPA. BPA is highly damaging to your cells. Even small amounts of BPAs cause damage to the entire cell. The water sits in hot warehouses and transport trucks, which cause further leaching of BPA.

If you are drinking out of plastic bottles that do not specifically say "BPA-free," then you are really risking your health. I live in "healthy" L.A. and have been able to find only one water company that makes BPA-free plastic. This most likely means you need to switch to reusable stainless-steel bottles with filtered water. Tap water would probably be a safer bet than drinking from BPA-made plastics.

BPA EXPOSURE = Damaged Mitochondria

A study published early in 2013 found that even small amounts of BPA exposure cause mitochondrial damage. The longer the exposure, the worse the damage; at 48 hours of exposure, even a small amount of BPA caused the mitochondria to lose function and increased the risk of the mitochondria membrane failing. Those damaged mitochondria were more likely to cause the cell to cannibalize itself and die.

If your cells aren't healthy enough to fight off or filter out toxins, your risk increases for developing:

- ✖ Fibroid cysts
- ✖ Fertility problems
- ✖ Birth defects
- ✖ Cancer
- ✖ Early Alzheimer's
- ✖ Autoimmune disorders
- ✖ Food allergies

These fat-soluble chemicals and other cell destroyers are sending your body into a daily red alert. Once stored, they undermine neural-cell function and alter memory, attention, alertness and mood.

Healthy cells can fight these everyday toxins, but crippled cells cannot. This is why we are seeing great numbers of people with intolerances to foods like gluten or dairy or an inability to eliminate poisons, such as mercury found in fish and seafood. Their cells have been overwhelmed by the constant chemical spill and simply can't react the way they're supposed to.

But there is a cure, and it starts with detoxifying your body's cells as much as you can. The next step is to provide your cells with the essential nutrients they need, and to adopt a lifestyle that helps feed your cells, not deplete them. You'll find that when your cells are happy, so are you!

I'm not asking you to live in a commune or rely on growing your own food, making your own clothing and giving up on any kind of hair or beauty product. That kind of extreme living wouldn't work for me, and it isn't realistic. You do have to realize that the cost of living in a toxic society is cellular damage and death, as well as the resulting diseases—unless you adopt a diet and lifestyle that will supercharge your cells and enable them to fight off today's toxins.

DANGEROUS DIETS

Improper dieting is a driving force behind deprived and broken-down cells. Despite repeatedly being proven in research to cause dysfunctions in energy, metabolism and mood, over 100 million people each year flock to the latest quick weight-loss fixes. Most will try to win the war against weight up to five times every year. This cycle of intermittent deprivation has proven not only to *prevent* weight loss but also to cause long-term bodily harm.

Many diet regimens focus on elimination and instruct individuals to cut out carbs, entire food groups or even solid foods altogether. I see the product of these kinds of programs all the time—people who come to me frustrated and fatigued from dieting. Their bodies have adapted, but every cell has been undernourished and can no longer function properly. Their systems are left in a state of emergency. They might even be thin from long-term deprivation, but they're dying on the inside. These "skinny fat" people are just as desperate for recovery as someone struggling with too much weight. Stay away from these fad diets:

- **LIQUID CLEANSES:** Fluid-only concoctions that promise a detoxifying effect, but have no proven benefits except temporary starvation. They're often dangerously low in calories and nutrients, and they cause your metabolism to permanently slow down, which leads to immediate weight gain when a more nutrient-dense diet is resumed.

- **NO-CARB DIETS:** Carbohydrates are the number-one source of fuel for muscles and the brain. Cut these out of your diet and your body will literally eat away its number-one defender against fat—muscle! When the body is forced to use muscle as fuel, it will be too weak to do much of anything besides basic bodily functions. Your drive and mood are severely negatively altered.

- **"UNI"-DIETS:** Diets that focus on eating only one type of food (like grapefruit or cabbage soup), which cause or deepen existing nutrient deficiencies, and create fatigue and mood imbalances.

As you can see, our bodies' cells are under attack every day from threats we cannot escape, even if we strive for a healthy lifestyle! Our cells are the body's building blocks, and when they start to malfunction, they impact other internal systems as well, as you'll see in the next chapter.

"WHEN YOU'RE BURNED OUT, YOU DON'T CARE ABOUT ANYTHING... **EXCEPT YOUR NEXT CRUTCH**"

CHAPTER TWO

BURN-OUT

SYNDROME:

THE REAL EPIDEMIC

**Seems like every day you hear someone on the news talking about the obesity epidemic. You'd have to be living under a rock not to know that we're the fattest country ever—and getting fatter by the day! We're fat. Our kids are fat. Their kids are going to be even fatter.
And, yeah, that's a huge health problem!**

But there's an epidemic that's just as dangerous that few people talk about—or are even aware of.

I'm talking about burnout. What I call burnout syndrome.

When you're burned out, you don't care about anything...except your next crutch. You're exhausted. You feel hopeless and helpless, as if there's no light at the end of the tunnel. You don't enjoy the things you used to.

Sounds like depression, doesn't it? Burnout syndrome does have a lot in common with depression, but it's even more common—and more insidious—than depression. It affects tens of millions of us, keeping us from having the energy and health we need to live our lives to the fullest.

Think about the last time you were struggling to meet a deadline at work, while dealing with a sick kid, a traveling spouse and your own lack of sleep. You felt stressed and may have struggled to juggle your responsibilities without crashing. Hopefully, things improved. You finished your project. Your kid got better. Your spouse came home. You got some sleep. The stressors you faced eased, at least temporarily.

When those stressors never let up, though, your body's stress response system gets overridden. You're unable to rise to the occasion, and you feel exhausted, overwhelmed and hopeless every day. That's burnout syndrome.

There are different kinds of exhaustion. You can be emotionally exhausted. You can be mentally exhausted. You can be physically exhausted. Burnout involves exhaustion of *all three systems*—emotional, mental and physical.

Symptoms of burnout syndrome include:

* Chronic/constant sense of fatigue
* Frequent illnesses (colds, asthma flare-ups, etc.)
* Muscle aches
* Headaches
* Back pain
* Lack of motivation to do anything—even your favorite hobbies
* A negative, bleak outlook
* Feeling hopeless and helpless, as if nothing will ever get better
* Feeling like a failure
* Feeling isolated from other people, even those you love
* Relying on overeating, alcohol or drugs to manage daily life
* Irritability
* Procrastination
* The sense that things will never improve

It's normal to feel some of these symptoms *some* of the time. When you feel like this all the time, though, or most of the time, it's a symptom of something far more serious than feeling stressed. It means that your body's glands are malfunctioning—the constant, unrelenting stress they're under is causing critical damage.

Each of us is biologically unique, and the conditions that cause one person to thrive will cause burnout syndrome in another. We think about stress as being a negative, but it isn't. Stress gets us out of bed in the morning. It helps get us through school, gets us to the gym when we'd rather skip a workout and makes us care about what people think of us. It makes us anxious before we speak in front of a group so that we perform better. It gives us the drive to be a better parent, a better partner, a better person. Without stress, we wouldn't have any drive, any get-up-and-go.

But even the most resilient of us isn't designed to be stressed all the time! Even our ancestors had periods of downtime when they didn't have to fight off a wild animal or compete for food. Their biological stress systems were able to reboot every night, and during the day when they weren't facing any acute stressors.

Today, we're subject to stressors 24/7. Our cell phones vibrate in the middle of the night. We drive in traffic with one hand on the wheel, one hand gripping a cup of coffee and an earbud in our ear. We multitask constantly without thinking about the consequences to our animal brains—and those consequences are dire.

"Information overload" is an increasing problem in today's society. On an average day, we're exposed to *12 hours' worth* of information at home—and that's not even counting what we experience at work. We're hooked on technology—everything from television to the internet and smartphones—and that's not good for our brains. Simply put, we cannot handle the amount of information thrown at us constantly, and there's always something new to learn, to master, to keep up with.

A new syndrome, called **"FOMO," or Fear of Missing Out**, is a real problem among teens and adults alike. We can't turn off our phones. We have to check our Twitter account. We must update our Facebook status. This constant connectivity means that our brains are always "on alert," which means our adrenals are, too. This leads to our bodies and brains being constantly awash in stress hormones, so it's not surprising that, according to the American Institute of Stress, 75–90 percent of doctors' visits are a direct result of stress.

Burnout syndrome can sneak up on you so gradually you don't even know you have it. It's so common it's become accepted as normal, but it's certainly not. Your body's cells are awesome but they weren't designed to handle all the toxins they're exposed to every day. They'll try to keep up, and do the best they can—but eventually they will fail.

That's what happens when you're burned out, too. The glands that control your body's response to stress—and keep you healthy, energetic, alert, focused and even attractive—are susceptible to day-in-day-out overuse. They get burned out, you get burned out and the cycle continues.

It sounds like a "chicken or egg" debate. Do you get burned out and then burn out your glands, or is it the other way around? I think it's a little bit of both. Let's look at what's happening on the inside of our bodies—at the glandular level.

THESE GLANDS HAVE HAD IT!

Burnout syndrome means your glands are burned out—or well on their way to being burned out. Your glands are like the boss of your energy—not quite the CEO that cells are, but just one step below. It's common in our culture to hear people blame weight gain on poor thyroid, and exhaustion on fatigued adrenals. If I had a dollar for every time I've heard someone say, "My adrenals are just wiped out!" I'd be a very rich woman.

Popular thought is that too much coffee is the primary enemy of adrenals, but there are many other factors within our control that cause glandular fatigue. Weight gain and exhaustion are due to a myriad of poor lifestyle choices, and those choices have a major impact on the glands that regulate metabolism and energy.

There are three vital glands that, when working well, keep the body running at its best and prevent burnout syndrome:

1 Pituitary gland (the so-called "master" gland)

2 Adrenal glands

3 Thyroid gland

I call these three the "beauty glands" because when we're healthy, they are responsible for many of the characteristics that make us look and feel attractive.

I can always spot a person with sickly glands. They are sallow and often look frazzled from everyday life.

These three vital glands are sensitive by design. Like fine instruments, they're tuned to sense shifts in energy, alertness and metabolism, and to trigger the precise hormonal disbursement required for every situation. Properly functioning glands create balanced moods and energy, help you sleep and give you great skin. The body is simply a bag of chemicals; your glands determine which chemical messages get released, and when, to keep your body functions balanced.

The good news is that healthy glands are completely within your control. However, these glands become depleted as a result of your daily habits and surprisingly toxic products. Here are some of the factors that cause gland dysfunction:

- ✖ A diet of processed foods (foods containing chemicals)
- ✖ Sugar substitutes
- ✖ Diet foods (fat-free and sugar-free foods)
- ✖ Excessive stress or worry
- ✖ Constant exposure to electronics
- ✖ Taking prescription and over-the-counter meds
- ✖ Drinking more than two glasses of alcohol a week
- ✖ Drinking three or more cups of coffee a day
- ✖ Smoking

As we saw in the last chapter, our cells are exposed to all kinds of toxins that didn't exist even 100 years ago. When our cells can't adapt to these poisons, cells malfunction and die. Well, our glands are no different in that they weren't designed for the stressors of the 21st century! They can be damaged by environmental factors, poor diet and unhealthy lifestyle choices—basically a stressed-out existence.

Overworked glands are telling you "enough is enough" by making you feel overwhelmed on a daily basis. There is a price to pay for living in a modern society and we gladly pay it, but we must have the antidote to the harm that it's causing. Let's take a look at these "boss" glands and their distinct roles in predicting energy and health deficiencies.

THE BIG 3

PITUITARY GLAND (MASTER GLAND)

The pituitary gland is a tiny gland located at the base of the brain. While it's small in size, it's called the "master gland" for a reason. This master gland governs the other hormone-secreting glands in the body, thereby controlling hormone function. Think of the pituitary as the foreman on a construction site (your body), giving commands to all his workers (adrenal/thyroid), as well as supplying enough materials for the job (hormones).

Hormones send important messages throughout the body. The pituitary releases five of the most critical hormones for health, happiness, vitality, beauty, sex drive and fertility. They are:

– HGH. Also known as human growth hormone, HGH regulates sugar and fat metabolism and promotes collagen growth. It is called the "youth hormone" because of its association with muscle growth, bone density, sex drive and skin rejuvenation.

– TSH. Thyroid-stimulating hormone is the hormone that turns on the production of two essential thyroid hormones—T3 and T4. As you'll see below, these hormones (in the right amount—not too little and not too much) are essential for metabolism, mood and energy.

– ACTH. Adrenocorticotrophic hormone is produced by the pituitary gland and stimulates the adrenal gland to produce cortisol, which maintains blood-glucose levels and helps your immune system function optimally.

– FSH/LH. Follicle-stimulating hormone and luteinizing hormone are produced by the pituitary gland and are essential for reproduction. In women, FSH and LH work together to stimulate ovulation; in men, they promote sperm production and increase testosterone.

The pituitary gland and the hormones it produces are susceptible to damage from chemicals called "endocrine disruptors." Endocrine disruptors literally scramble and confuse the natural communication of hormones, interfering with how the body is supposed to work. These chemicals tend to accumulate in fat cells and are not excreted by the body. Having a defense against these toxins is crucial.

Endocrine disruptors include:

✖ Fluoride. In the 1950s, communities started adding fluoride to their water supplies to help reduce cavities, and now about two-thirds of Americans have access to fluoridated water. While this (along with fluoride-containing toothpaste and better dental care overall) has helped reduce the amount of tooth decay in the population, studies show that fluoride accumulates in the pineal gland, affecting melatonin production, an essential hormone that helps you sleep.

✖ Bisphenol A. As you read in chapter 1, BPA is found in everything from water bottles to food cans to water-supply pipes to compact discs, and interferes with normal hormone production.

✖ Pharmaceuticals. Some drugs, including oral contraceptives and hormone replacement therapy, are designed to mimic natural hormones and are endocrine disruptors. Even if you don't take these drugs, they get into the water supply and you wind up drinking them without even knowing.

✖ Polychlorinated biphenyls. Also known as PCBs, these chemicals have been used in everything from paint, dyes, plastics and rubber products to electrical and hydraulic equipment. They are known carcinogens, or cancer-causers, in addition to endocrine disruptors.

✖ Mold. Mold is a type of fungus that grows both outdoors and indoors, and many people are sensitive to it. Symptoms of mold exposure include wheezing, stuffiness, eye irritation and skin irritation. Exposure to mold can also interfere with pituitary gland function. If you have breathing issues that don't go away, or get worse during the winter (when you're inside more often), I suggest you have your home inspected for mold.

✖ **Mercury from fillings.** While this metal is known to be poisonous, it has long been used in dental fillings. Ask your dentist to check the integrity of your old fillings and to always give you a gold or composite filling.

Endocrine disruptors are found in everyday products that may surprise you, including:

✖ Plastic bottles

✖ Metal food cans

✖ Detergents

✖ Air fresheners

✖ Flame retardants

✖ Boxed food

✖ Toys

✖ Cosmetics

We've looked at some of the environmental factors that can affect your pituitary gland. Now let's look at some of the bad dietary choices that can cause pituitary damage.

✖ **Processed foods (foods with added chemicals).** A diet that is high in processed food produces free radicals, which attack the cells of your pituitary gland.

✖ **Mercury from fish.** Fish that swim in polluted waters are high in endocrine disruptors; in general, the larger the fish, the more mercury it contains. Children and fetuses are particularly vulnerable to mercury, and pregnant women are told to avoid fish such as king mackerel, shark, swordfish and tilefish, which have the highest mercury levels. Other fish that have high levels of mercury and other toxins include grouper, halibut, orange roughy and tuna steaks (canned tuna tends to have less mercury).

✖ **Nonorganically grown meat.** Endocrine disruptors are stored in the fat of animals and humans alike, so consuming meat and poultry that have been exposed to pesticides and herbicides means that you're consuming pituitary toxins as well.

✖ **GMOs.** *GMOs* sound better than what these foods are really called— genetically modified organisms. What? Don't sound so tasty, do they? Genetically modified (or genetically engineered foods) have been selectively developed by taking the genes of a plant (or animal) and placing them into another organism. Common foods such as corn, potatoes, squash, soybeans and tomatoes have all been genetically modified in the United States; most are used to make ingredients used in processed foods. These "foods" have been touted as a way to feed more people, and their dangers have been downplayed. But in addition to causing tumors, organ failure, liver damage and allergic reactions, eating GMOs can disrupt your hormone function as well.

Symptoms of pituitary gland dysfunction depend on what hormones are affected, and how much (or how little) of them are produced. Because the pituitary gland controls the adrenal and thyroid glands, the symptoms of pituitary dysfunction resemble those of adrenal and thyroid dysfunction, which I'll discuss in more detail in the sections below. But in general, those symptoms include:

- ✖ Low sex drive
- ✖ Fertility problems
- ✖ Hair loss
- ✖ Anxious/nervous feelings

- ✖ Racing heartbeat
- ✖ Unexplained weight loss or weight gain
- ✖ Inflammation
- ✖ High blood sugar

Getting this master gland healthy is key because of its control over two other glands that play a major role in your health:

- – Thyroid, which controls metabolism
- – Adrenal, which helps our bodies respond to stress

If the pituitary is working well, it releases appropriate amounts of hormones that keep you at a healthy weight, keep you in a good mood and maintain a healthy sex drive. This program includes specific foods that contain the essential nutrients that stimulate the pituitary to maintain healthy hormone levels—and help keep the adrenal and thyroid glands functioning optimally, too.

ADRENAL GLANDS (ENERGY GLANDS)

The adrenal glands are located right above the kidneys and they look like a small bag of marbles. When they're imbalanced or fatigued, we're pushed to extremes, swinging from tired and unmotivated to agitated and anxious, constantly on edge.

Adrenals work hard to maintain:

1 Appropriate stress responses

2 Fat storage and energy production

3 Immune response

When you're burned out, your adrenals are burned out, too. And when the adrenals are burned out, every organ in your body is negatively impacted.

When your adrenals are exhausted, basically you look crappy, feel crappy and then stay anxious about how you look and feel—which causes more adrenal fatigue. It's an endless, exhausting loop.

EXHAUSTED ADRENALS = A Sad and Tired You

Adrenal burnout can be caused by:

* ✖ Stressful home, school or work environments
* ✖ A major life change that causes fear or trepidation
* ✖ A chronic infection such as the flu or bronchitis
* ✖ A tumultuous relationship with your family or partner

People with adrenal fatigue have a hard time managing stress. They feel constantly overwhelmed, constantly depressed and constantly forgetful. No wonder they have sleep problems and struggle to get out of bed in the morning!

Adrenal exhaustion affects fertility so if you are trying to get pregnant, it's time to get your adrenals healthy.

The adrenal glands are the first level of defense, the "Secret Service" of your body. They leap into action to help you physically and mentally keep your cool in times of distress. The short-term side effects of adrenal fatigue are uncomfortable but not intolerable. It's believed that 80 percent of the population suffers from adrenal fatigue in varying degrees. Yes, you can drag yourself out of bed, drink lots of coffee and manage anxiety by constantly checking your phone, but your mood and sense of well-being will be greatly compromised.

You may be amazed at how many conditions you accept as "normal" that are actually signs of adrenal fatigue. One of the most common symptoms is fatigue that is unrelieved by sleep; you go to bed tired and you wake up tired. Feeling constantly overwhelmed or unable to cope with your everyday demands is another symptom. If you find yourself getting angry over every little thing or being driven to tears over a minor insecurity or disagreement, chances are your adrenals are shot.

Let's break down the symptoms of adrenal burnout into two categories—physical and emotional:

PHYSICAL

✖ Sleep disturbances	✖ Muscle weakness
✖ Intense cravings for sweets and coffee	✖ Chronic cough, asthma or bronchitis
✖ Addictive behavior	✖ Allergies
✖ Continual sickness/infections	✖ Headaches
✖ Frequent urination and thirst	✖ Varicose veins/hemorrhoids
✖ Dizziness	✖ Heart palpitations

EMOTIONAL

- ✖ Feeling run-down or overwhelmed
- ✖ Feeling like you are a "pressure cooker" ready to burst
- ✖ Difficulty handling/bouncing back from stress
- ✖ Panic attacks

- ✖ Feeling more awake, alert and energetic after 6:00 p.m. than you do all day
- ✖ Depression/anxiety
- ✖ Feelings of dread or persecution
- ✖ Mind fog/memory problems

Your adrenal glands are designed to handle any type of stress you're exposed to, but they can't be on "high alert" forever. Until fairly recently, the job of our adrenal glands was fairly simple. They responded to occasional "calls to action," like outrunning a predator or simply responding in the face of occasional high stress.

In this modern age, however, we are consistently under stress—dealing with financial crises, trying to find and keep a job, juggling a career and a family, and the constant bombardment of advertising and information. Our adrenals are finely tuned instruments, but they weren't meant for the Information Age we live in today.

Our adrenals are never "off the clock." Our stress today is chronic and unrelenting, causing these tiny glands to constantly be "on"; they simply can't keep up with the demand. As a result, they become unable to function properly, and can't play their other role in balancing the other hormones such as norepinephrine (adrenaline), cortisol and DHEA that are essential for health. I've given you the "big picture" about what happens when your adrenals are kaput, but here are three specific conditions that a malfunctioning adrenal will cause.

CORTISOL FLOODING

Cortisol mobilizes nutrients, enables the body to fight inflammation and increases energy. When balanced, cortisol stimulates the storage and release of energy in the body, helps the body resist the stressful effects of infections and trauma, and helps you maintain stable emotions.

Unfortunately, there can be too much of a good thing. When the adrenal glands release too much cortisol in response to stress, it can result in:

- ✖ A weakened immune system
- ✖ Constant anxiety that leads to fear and depression
- ✖ Stubborn weight gain
- ✖ An inability to lose weight
- ✖ Loss of bone density
- ✖ An inability to tone muscle
- ✖ Thinning of the skin, causing wrinkles and dark under-eye circles
- ✖ Kidney damage/frequent urination
- ✖ Food and environmental allergies
- ✖ Cancer

It's important to remember that while your brain may know that something isn't really a threat, your "animal brain" does not. So while you can tell yourself, "It's okay—don't get stressed," you're never completely able to avoid stressors. Your adrenal glands are designed to respond to and cope with stress, but when the stress becomes unrelenting they go awry.

DHEA DROP

DHEA is another hormone produced by your adrenal glands. It has anti-aging effects and is essential for good health; low levels of DHEA have been linked with an array of conditions, including cancer, cardiovascular disease, Alzheimer's, diabetes, depression, hypothyroidism and adrenal fatigue. It's called a "sex hormone" because it's necessary to produce testosterone and estrogen, which affect sex drive and fertility. DHEA works in conjunction with cortisol; when DHEA goes up, cortisol goes down and vice versa. It also keeps cortisol in check by neutralizing its immunosuppressant effect.

It's not the amount of DHEA that we worry about, but the ratio of cortisol to DHEA in your body. That ratio is constantly in flux, depending on what's happening in your body, but when DHEA drops too low, you may experience:

- ✖ Slow recovery from illness
- ✖ High cholesterol
- ✖ Insomnia
- ✖ Low sex drive
- ✖ Fertility problems
- ✖ Fatigue
- ✖ Foggy brain
- ✖ An inability to recover from stressful situations

Because DHEA is produced by your adrenals, malfunctioning adrenals interfere with its production, and make you more likely to experience the above symptoms. DHEA levels also start to drop in your 30s. Because it's essential for the production of sex hormones, a low sex drive is often a sign of a lack of this critical hormone. DHEA supplements are common but a better approach is to balance your DHEA levels by supporting your adrenal gland function.

ADRENALINE SURGE AND STORAGE

Adrenaline is commonly thought of as the fight-or-flight hormone. It can work well to manage stress and give us an edge in athletics, social situations or work performance. When released during exercise, it gives us more energy, makes us better coordinated and gives us the drive to finish a challenging workout. When we're not working out, though, our body lacks an outlet for that adrenaline, and we feel anxious, nauseous, shaky or weak until adrenaline levels drop.

When you feel threatened, an adrenaline surge is released that will make your heart pound, your brain grow sharper and your pain tolerance rise. Typically, we don't experience a life-threatening event on a regular basis, making an adrenaline surge useful. Instead, something more insidious occurs—a constant and continuous tension and stress that cause a buildup but do not allow a release of adrenaline. Our bodies remain on high alert and cause us harm. Some of the symptoms related to adrenaline surge and storage include:

- ✳ Insomnia
- ✳ Anxiety
- ✳ Paranoia
- ✳ Reactivity/quickness to anger

- ✳ Inability to concentrate or organize thoughts
- ✳ Social awkwardness/ nervousness
- ✳ Lowered immunity

Your body's adrenaline is like a power booster button you can push when you need some extra get-up-and-go. It gives you the drive to face modern-day challenges, like getting off the couch and exercising, and it promotes lifesaving reactions like swerving suddenly to avoid a texting driver who's about to collide with you. Persistent stress causes a continual release of adrenaline that keeps you in an anxious flight-or-flight mode throughout your day. This chemical buildup leads to the depletion of adrenals.

Historically, adrenaline surged to prepare us for battle or to perform some sort of lifesaving activity. Now, we have daily surges as a result of feeling consistently overwhelmed as a result of work stressors, financial stressors and interpersonal relationships—basically from being alive at this time. Think of these adrenaline surges as withdrawals from a bank to help you get through life's rough spots. If you get into the habit of withdrawing adrenaline from your account too often, you'll eventually be overdrawn and your adrenal glands will be overwhelmed. Then you won't be able to "power up" when you really need to.

Without adrenaline, you wouldn't be able to respond to life crises both big and small, but you can't rely on its power forever. Think of it as an occasional boost, not your regular energy source. The more you use it, the less you'll have of it when you really need it.

DAILY DRAINS

Chances are your daily life is stressing your adrenals, but you may be making matters worse if you're exposed to any of these daily drains:

- ✳ **Three or more cups of coffee.** Caffeine stimulates your central nervous system, making you feel more alert. It's also proven to improve your brain function in small doses, but experts say that you shouldn't consume more than about 200 milligrams of caffeine (about two cups of coffee) a day. Drinking three or more cups of coffee overstimulates your nervous system and creates a minor fight-or-flight response that your adrenal glands have to address.

* **Supercharged energy drinks.** These contain caffeine and other stimulants that have the same impact on your central nervous system, amping you up. These drinks (Red Bull, 5-Hour Energy and Monster) contain anywhere from 80 to 240 milligrams of caffeine, far more than soda, which clocks in at about 35 milligrams for 12 ounces.

* **Fast foods and processed foods.** These foods contain additives, GMOs and chemicals that can throw off your adrenal glands' function.

* **Drinking too little.** As you've learned, exhausted adrenals lead to chronic dehydration. Two to three liters of water daily is optimal for energy and organ detox.

* **"Natural" energy-producing supplements.** Supplements that contain ingredients such as guarana and green tea artificially amp you up, and will further throw your body's hormone balance out of whack.

* **Synthetic drugs.** Your body isn't able to metabolize all human-made compounds such as manufactured drugs, and taking them can interfere with adrenal function.

* **Eating a lot of sugar.** Foods high in sugar send your blood glucose levels into overdrive, artificially amping you up like an energy drink. High-sugar foods turn on your body's cortisol production, artificially stimulating your adrenal gland to make more.

* **Too much screen time.** There's a good chance that you spend at least eight hours a day—likely more—staring at a screen. When you're always watching television, staring at a computer screen or on your smartphone, you're constantly stimulating your senses, your brain and your adrenal glands.

I wouldn't be telling you all these scary facts if I didn't have a concrete solution to offer you. The adrenals are very resilient and in a short amount of time can be altered and made healthier. Adrenal fatigue may be the norm, but that doesn't mean you have to settle for it!

My program will help you overcome adrenal burnout and help your adrenals function the way they're supposed to—responding appropriately, not melodramatically—and you'll feel worlds better as a result.

THYROID GLAND (METABOLISM MASTER)

We hear more about adrenal fatigue than thyroid fatigue, but the thyroid is a very important gland for energy, weight control, beauty and positive mood. The thyroid gland is shaped like a butterfly and is located in the lower part of the neck, wrapped around the windpipe. While the adrenals respond to danger like highly tuned bodyguards, the thyroid gland does the everyday work of a manager. Your thyroid determines, among other things, how fast you burn calories, how fast your heart beats and how fast you digest food.

Thyroid hormones affect everything from your body's internal temperature to your weight, the strength of your muscles, your skin's suppleness and your breathing. Even your brain, your heart and cardiovascular system, and your nervous system respond to your thyroid's commands.

In regard to the body, science is frequently left asking, "Which comes first, the chicken or the egg?" Dysfunction of a gland like the thyroid, for example, is rarely generated by that gland. One organ or imbalance of chemicals will adversely affect another, causing diagnosis to be very difficult. Most of your thyroid hormone conversion happens in the liver. If your liver is overworked trying to process medications, caffeine, alcohol, food chemicals and sugar, most likely your thyroid function is going haywire.

Yet standard blood tests will detect only major dysfunctions when the thyroid gland is the source of the problem and won't tell you when it's just subpar. An impaired cellular transport system—due to sick cells, as explained in the last chapter—also negatively affects the thyroid. This program will

will thoroughly heal cells so that they can send the right chemical messages to the thyroid.

The thyroid uses iron and iodine to make three key hormones:

- Thyroxin (T4). T4 is the main thyroid hormone; your body produces about four times more T4 than T3. The job of T4 is simple—to produce T3.

- Triiodothyronine (T3). T4 produces T3, but your thyroid also produces T3 directly. This hormone affects metabolic rate, macronutrient turnover, and vitamin and mineral absorption. While your body produces much less T3, this hormone is much more active than T4 and is responsible for boosting metabolism by increasing the number of calories you use at rest, what's called your "basal metabolism." T3 also is used to break down protein and carbohydrates, and to remove unhealthy cholesterol from your blood.

- Calcitonin. This hormone stimulates bone cells to add calcium to bone. Calcitonin, along with parathyroid hormone, works to regulate the amount of calcium circulating in your blood. While you probably think of calcium as being something you consume to make strong bones, this mineral is also essential for cellular function and for your nervous system.

A malfunctioning thyroid can do one of two things—produce too much of particular hormones or produce too little. Both states have similar negative effects on the body, making you uncomfortable and unhealthy. It's estimated that up to 60 million people in the United States have hypothyroidism or hyperthyroidism, but this figure may not even take into account the people who don't meet the clinical definition of either condition yet suffer from a surplus or a lack of these powerful hormones.

ANXIOUS AND PARANOID: HYPERTHYROID

A hyperactive thyroid is like a hopped-up manager; instead of taking care of the basic needs, it's jumping here and there and interfering with your body's normal processes. Your thyroid is in overdrive, so your body is revved up all the time, leading to a slew of health problems.

One of the most commonly noticed signs of an overactive thyroid is a too-fast, or irregular, heartbeat. Your metabolism is amped up, and you can feel it; you may notice your heart pounding or that you're constantly short of breath and breathing hard even when you're taking it easy. This jacked-up metabolism often makes you feel nervous, anxious, and weak or exhausted, and you can't figure out why.

Think of how you feel when you're nervous, such as preparing to give a speech to a group of people. An overactive thyroid makes you feel like that *all the time*. You feel shaky, weak and sweaty; your hands may shake; you may feel anxious and upset for no apparent reason. Because your metabolism is operating at such a high level, you may lose weight without changing your diet, and may have diarrhea or notice that you're constantly in the bathroom.

Too much thyroid hormone can also interfere with cholesterol metabolism, causing levels of blood cholesterol to plummet. While cholesterol is given a bad rap, it's essential for brain function, for the production of sex hormones and for cellular communication. Too little of it is linked with depression, anxiety, suicide attempts, impulsivity and aggressive behavior.

You're likely to see the effects of an overactive thyroid in the mirror, too. High thyroid hormone levels mean that fatty acids (produced when fats break down) increase, glucose is more easily stored in cells and protein degrades, which can lead to faster growing but brittle, easily broken nails and thin hair that falls out easily.

And finally, your level of thyroid-stimulating hormone, which turns on the production of the other three hormones, is linked with fertility; if it's too high, it impairs your ability to get pregnant. It may also interfere with your menstrual cycle and prevent ovulation, which causes menstrual irregularities that make it harder to conceive.

Symptoms of an overactive thyroid include:

- ✖ Increased heart rate
- ✖ Anxiety or panic attacks
- ✖ Diarrhea or irritable bowel syndrome (IBS)
- ✖ Unhealthily low cholesterol levels (total cholesterol levels of less than 160 mg/dL)
- ✖ Shorter, lighter or infrequent menstruation
- ✖ Nervousness/social awkwardness
- ✖ Irritability
- ✖ Poor nail and hair quality
- ✖ Thin, crepey skin

FAT AND TIRED: HYPOTHYROID

Then there's the thyroid that is not producing enough thyroid hormones, causing hypothyroidism. This is the lazy manager; the manager who can't be bothered to get up from his desk and actually do what he's supposed to do. That means that your body's metabolism is sluggish, which causes a slew of symptoms.

> " AN INABILITY TO LOSE AND KEEP OFF WEIGHT, EVEN ON A DIET AND EXERCISE PROGRAM, IS **ANOTHER SIGN OF THYROID MALFUNCTION** "

One of the major symptoms is unrelenting fatigue. With hypothyroidism, you're hyped up but also exhausted because your metabolism is in overdrive. With too few thyroid hormones, though, you just feel spent all the time. You're tired when you wake up. You're tired during the day. You're tired at night. And then the cycle repeats itself.

An inability to lose and keep off weight, even on a diet and exercise program, is another sign of thyroid malfunction. Thyroid malfunction can interfere with even the most dedicated dieter's plans. It depresses your metabolism so that you're burning fewer calories all the time, making it nearly impossible to lose weight.

Remember that the amount of calories you burn through exercise is minimal compared to how much your body burns the rest of the time, called your basal metabolism. If your basal metabolism is depressed, you'll burn fewer calories all the time, regardless of your activity level or diet—and if you overeat, you'll store more of that extra food as fat.

In addition to fatigue, you may notice that your muscles feel achy or tender, or that your joints are stiff and sore. Your hair may thin and/or fall out, and you may find it hard to focus or concentrate. You may feel depressed much of the time. Because your metabolism is sluggish, you may also feel colder than usual, even in a warm room. Your skin may be dry and flaky, you may be constipated and you may gain weight without changing your diet or activity level.

A thyroid that's exhausted may produce the following symptoms:

- ✖ Muscle and joint pains/carpal tunnel syndrome/tendonitis
- ✖ Fatigue, insomnia and daytime exhaustion
- ✖ Brain fog/poor memory
- ✖ Weight problems
- ✖ Depression
- ✖ Poor hair and/or skin quality
- ✖ Constipation
- ✖ High cholesterol that doesn't respond to diet
- ✖ Irregular menstruation/fertility problems

These are all symptoms of thyroid malfunction; your thyroid isn't managing your body's systems aggressively enough (remember our lazy manager) and you'll have a hard time feeling enthusiastic or energetic about anything. Thyroid disease tends to creep up on you slowly, though, so you may not even notice that you're gradually feeling more tired, more depressed, more achy. It's only when you look back and realize you haven't always felt this way that you may sense something is wrong.

DAILY DRAINS

Major stress, empty calories and poor sleep quality can cause a severe imbalance of the thyroid and the systems affecting hormone production. The thyroid is also affected by triggers such as chronic illness, inflammation, depression, obesity and insulin imbalance. All these ailments and symptoms will be greatly and positively affected by this program. The scary truth is that the thyroid is like a target for toxins. Here are just a few that affect your thyroid:

- Triclosan, found in toothpastes and antibacterial soaps, has been proven to disrupt thyroid function.
- Phthalates, used in plastics and fragrances, suppress thyroid hormones in men and affect fertility.
- Perchlorate, which is found in soil and some fertilizers, is a well-known thyroid disruptor. This chemical has been found in significant levels in water systems, and has contaminated groundwater in the western United States.
- BPAs, which are found in plastic and are particularly dangerous in water bottles.
- PCBs. These chemicals are not easily broken down so we're constantly exposed to them; experts say that there are 1.5 million metric tons of PCBs spread over the surface of the earth. You wind up consuming these chemicals when you eat meat, poultry, fish and dairy products produced by animals that have been exposed them as well. (This is another reason to eat free-range and organic.)

It's highly unrealistic to presume that you will stop using all products that are toxic. What do you do when the very soil and water that you get your foods from are poisoning you? I'm not asking you to join a commune or stop brushing your teeth. To live is to be slightly toxic, but there is a defense against these environmental factors.

The minerals and nutrients that you will consume in this diet will be a tonic for your wounded glands—your pituitary, adrenals and thyroid. All of life's stressors—and the havoc they wreak—can be managed by easy lifestyle changes so that you can begin looking and feeling your best.

DANGEROUS DRUGS

The increase in thyroid issues, which are 50 percent more likely to hit women than men, shouldn't signal the need for synthetic intervention. In fact, synthetic hormones can shut down your body's natural production of thyroid hormones, and create a lifetime need. Good for the pharmaceutical industry, bad for you. However, doctors typically suggest you pop a pill instead of addressing the underlying issues of *why* your thyroid isn't working right!

If your body relies on an artificial source of hormone—the synthetic hormone in drugs—it has no reason to get its body manager back in line, so to speak. This means you're stuck taking thyroid medication for the rest of your life.

Yet the opposite can happen, too. Taking drugs for hypothyroidism may overstimulate the thyroid and cause hyperthyroidism. You then constantly have to change the dose of your drug while you still suffer from symptoms of a thyroid that's out of whack.

The smarter choice is to protect your thyroid by making changes in the way you live and stay off the drug train forever.

You've seen how bodies' glands interact with each other, and are often disrupted, not only by what we put in our bodies, but by what our bodies are exposed to. In a cleaner, less toxic environment, our glandular systems and the other systems of the body function smoothly, but it's clear that our daily lives are loaded with substances that throw these essential systems off-kilter. There's one more powerful factor at play as well—something we often disregard at our peril. It's how we sleep.

"ONE NIGHT OF POOR SLEEP WILL SET THE DAMAGE IN MOTION **AND MOST DEFINITELY RUIN YOUR DAY**"

CHAPTER THREE

POOR SLEEP:

THE SILENT KILLER

More than 70 million Americans suffer from sleep problems. Most experience nagging to severe side effects, but don't identify repeated restless nights as the cause. Even science is just starting to catch on to the wide net poor-quality sleep casts across human health. Recent research has revealed the crucial link between sleep deprivation and the body's inability to fight disease and sickness. Poor sleep is crippling our immune systems and contributing to an epidemic of autoimmune disorders such as psoriasis, fibromyalgia, chronic fatigue syndrome and rheumatoid arthritis.

Lost sleep leads to dramatic dysfunction in blood sugar levels, metabolism, mood, memory and immunity. Emotional stability is particularly affected, with research revealing that six hours of sleep or fewer per night can disrupt parts of the brain linked to depression and other mental disorders. It might take years for these serious conditions to develop, but even one night of poor sleep will set the damage in motion and most definitely ruin your day.

Sleep deprivation makes you spend your days in a literal daze, feeling forgetful, out of sorts and out of touch with reality. Emotions can go haywire, leading to an inability to judge situations appropriately, and wreaking havoc on personal and business relationships. Lost productivity, failed relationships and a hostile temperament toward others and the world are some of the symptoms of sleep disruption.

Your essential appetite hormones—leptin and ghrelin—will be a mess from sleep deprivation, too. They stop signaling properly, paving the way for uncontrollable weight gain. Additionally, low-quality sleep can damage DNA and increase oxidative stress, setting up an environment where cancer can thrive. Research shows that just one week of shortened sleep times altered 856 genes, many of which are imperative to immune health, stress management, inflammation response and fertility. This DNA damage can become permanent and be passed on to any future children you have.

The bottom line is that too little shut-eye doesn't just create sleepiness; it leads to a deep level of dysfunction within systems that control immunity, metabolism and mood. These dysfunctions go on to make you sick, tired, depressed and unable to lose weight. The average adult *should* be getting between seven-and-a-half and nine hours of sleep a night. These days, getting less than seven hours a night is commonplace, and plenty of people try to run on five hours or fewer. The difference between seven and seven and a half hours is significant, since the skipped minutes were most likely intended to be essential REM sleep. As these hours of lost sleep build up over time—days, weeks, years—a "sleep debt" is created. In this case, the deficit leaves you trying to function on nothing but fumes.

If you continue to take shortcuts on sleep, you're putting your health, happiness and life in danger. Chronic sleep loss is linked to the following:

- ✖ Higher risk for developing chronic anxiety and full-blown depression
- ✖ Greater risk for developing aggressive breast cancer, and prostate, endometrial and colon cancers
- ✖ Four times the risk for stroke
- ✖ Nearly twice the risk for diabetes and heart attack
- ✖ Permanent short-term memory loss
- ✖ Increased "brain plaque"—a precursor to Alzheimer's
- ✖ Twice the risk for dementia

THE SECRET LIFE OF SLEEP

You may not know it, but each night after you close your eyes, your brain and body put on a brilliantly choreographed performance designed to produce the best version of you each morning. Your sleep performance should include three acts, or stages: light sleep, deep sleep and dream sleep (or REM sleep). Sleep experts divide these stages into four non-REM stages and the REM stage for five different "types" of sleep. In healthy sleep, these will happen consecutively, completing a cycle in about 90 minutes and then repeating. If you wake up feeling refreshed, you've probably gone through the cycle five times, the optimal number of cycles for health and energy.

In *light sleep*, first your muscles twitch and you might hallucinate a ringing phone or someone calling your name. In stage 1 sleep, you're easily awakened because you're between wakefulness and sleep. Then, as you enter stage 2 sleep, your heart rate begins to slow and your body temperature decreases as you disconnect from your surroundings. This stage acts like a shuttle, transporting you to the more important later stages—but you can't get to your dream destination without getting on here first.

Stages 3 and 4 are where deep sleep occurs. During *deep sleep*, slow brain waves, called delta waves, occur and your muscles are deactivated for systemwide maintenance. Blood flow to your muscles increases. Deep sleep is the most vital for body repair—it's during this stage that growth hormone (GH) is pulsed into the body, where it renews skin and muscle tissue, builds bone, stimulates new cells and rejuvenates vital organs. Nearly 80 percent of GH is produced in deep sleep. The immune-cell messengers tumor necrosis factor (TNF) and interleukin-1beta (IL) also rise here, pushing you deeper into sleep so they can fix wounds and infections, and kill off bad cells.

Missing out on deep sleep will speed up aging, increase your risk for getting everything from colds to cancer and weaken your muscles. Drinking wine or downing cocktails before bed prevents you from getting into this deep sleep stage. You might pass out when you hit the pillow, but restorative sleep will be disrupted and once it is, your GH production shuts down.

About 90 minutes after you fall asleep, your body enters its first stage of REM sleep. In *dream sleep*, the brain becomes highly active and the eyes move rapidly and randomly, giving this stage its name of rapid-eye movement (REM) sleep. Here, the brain shelves important memories, trashes unwanted ones and works through vivid dreams.

Dream sleep is key to well-being because this is where your brain processes traumas and fears in a safe, unconscious way. Without this time of categorizing and cleanup, you would be a frightened, neurotic mess in your waking hours; in your dreams tonight, you create tomorrow's mood. Emotional balance is a delicate thing, and research shows that in dream sleep, we stitch together the stability of our sense of self. Dream sleep gets progressively longer and deeper with each sleep cycle, which is why, when you first wake up, you'll often remember bits and pieces of a fresh dream.

THE CHEMICAL CLOCK

Sleep happens as a result of hundreds of hormonal adjustments—those that wake you up have to be turned off, and those that create sleep have to be turned on. These hormones are highly sensitive to sound, smell, touch, hunger, stress and especially to light. Many everyday habits disrupt hormone timing, leading to lost sleep and weight gain, and put people in a constantly agitated and edgy state. Three primary hormones play an active role in sleep—cortisol, progesterone and prolactin.

CORTISOL

This hormone originates in the fight-or-flight response and is intended to help you react to danger. When we were nomadic and living in the wilderness, cortisol increased our chances of survival, boosting fuel to the blood and brain so we could think and act quickly in the face of a predator. Now, it gets constantly released in response to threat number one: stress. You can imagine that it's hard to fall or stay asleep when you're in fight-or-flight mode all night! By design, cortisol should simmer down after the initial response to a stressful situation and be practically nonexistent by evening, when you're ready for sleep.

But when you combine lots of stress and too little sleep, the feedback loop that produces cortisol gets jammed and you end up with chronically high levels of this hormone. Less than one week of shortened sleep can cause the body to produce cortisol six times slower. High cortisol levels will disrupt sleep, cause weight gain, make you more prone to illness, stall thinking and memory functions, weaken muscles, cause blood sugar chaos and damage your looks (science links high cortisol to lowered attractiveness). Loneliness and isolation also have proven links to high cortisol. When your body constantly signals for more cortisol to be produced, you end up low in progesterone, another hormone important to sleep.

PROGESTERONE

Progesterone is a steroid hormone that acts like a sedative when it comes to sleep: when it's balanced, sleep comes easily. Progesterone also helps regulate the thyroid, governs immune health, strengthens muscle tissue, stimulates collagen production and determines fertility in women. However, when the need for cortisol is high, a "progesterone steal" happens—the body grabs up all the pregnenolone (a progesterone precursor) it needs to make cortisol first before producing any other important hormones like progesterone. This system of prioritizing might have been helpful when danger was present, but in modern times the combination of high cortisol and low progesterone leads to anxiety, infertility, disrupted sleep and a seriously damaged quality of life.

PROLACTIN

This hormone is known for its role in breast health, but it performs nearly 300 other important jobs in the body. Chemically similar to growth hormone, it helps repair tissues and cells, and controls immune responses. Prolactin is released during deep sleep and promotes uninterrupted deep and dream sleep. Working in just the opposite way of cortisol, prolactin levels should surge at night and drop during the day. High levels are linked to decreased progesterone, anxiety, hypothyroidism, lowered sex hormones, infertility, erectile dysfunction, increased food intake and weight gain. Your daily habits have a big effect on prolactin: BPA, heavy metals, antihistamines, birth control pills, antidepressants, blood pressure medications and stress can all interfere with prolactin production.

"THE LESS YOU SLEEP,
**THE MORE LIKELY
YOU ARE TO BE FAT** "

Constant sleep deprivation and interruption of sleep cycles lead to a harsh but real outcome. You will increasingly become less mentally sharp, fatter, sicker and less stable in managing your moods. Let's look at how this works.

LACK OF SLEEP MAKES YOU STUPID

Even one night's worth of poor sleep affects your performance the next day, making it harder to stay alert and pay attention. Yes, part of this is due to fatigue, but there are other, more insidious factors at work, too. Remember that normally during sleep your body's cortisol levels drop, to rise again the next morning. Well, when you don't sleep enough, you don't experience this drop. Your level of cortisol—one of the hormones that hops you up—is already high and climbs even higher when you awaken. You wouldn't try to make a critical decision while you were swerving in traffic, would you? That high blood cortisol makes it all but impossible to focus, concentrate and learn. It's "brain fog" that can continue day after day.

Second, memories are organized and stored during REM sleep, and interrupting that makes it harder to remember not only what you ate for lunch the day before, but also the password to your online bank account or how to use a new computer program. Loss of sleep impacts both your short-term and long-term memory, and makes you more likely to develop Alzheimer's disease.

That loss of memory also impairs your judgment. Not only are you unable to think clearly, you can't compare your options to what's happened in the past or assess the pros and cons of any given situation at work and at home. This makes you a subpar parent, partner and person!

It's one thing to joke about being unable to recall someone's name or misplacing your keys, but lack of sleep hurts you at work—and might get you fired. And I don't even want to imagine what could happen if you have a job where a mistake could cost people their lives—sleep deprivation is a leading cause of medical errors, which kill 100,000 people a year. Fall asleep behind the wheel and you may never wake up—more than one-third of people admit to falling asleep while driving and experts now say that one in five accidents is the result of "drowsy" driving.

LACK OF SLEEP MAKES YOU FAT

I'll keep it simple for you. The less you sleep, the more likely you are to be fat. Sleep fewer than 6 hours a night and you are *7.5 times* more likely to be overweight than people who sleep at least 7.7 hours a night.

Lack of sleep reduces the level of leptin, a hormone that suppresses appetite, and increases ghrelin, a peptide produced by the stomach, which stimulates appetite. During normal sleep, leptin increases and ghrelin rises at first, and then decreases during the second half of sleep. Well, when you don't get enough sleep, the opposite happens: leptin levels plummet and ghrelin skyrockets. One study found that just two nights of four-hour sleep produced an 18 percent decrease in leptin, a 28 percent increase in ghrelin and a 24 percent increase in hunger, including a 32 percent increase in appetite for high-carbohydrate foods! Over time, these chemicals get more and more out of whack, and you get hungrier, eat more and get fat—or fatter.

Over the past fifty years, people's sleep average has dropped from 8 to 8.9 hours to about 7 hours a night. At the same time, the rates of obesity and type 2 diabetes have skyrocketed. Coincidence? I don't think so.

But obesity isn't only bad for your health. Bottom line: when you're fat—especially when you're obese—you don't feel good about yourself. I've never met someone who was significantly overweight and truly happy. Being overweight is linked to poor self-esteem and higher rates of depression and anxiety.

Most overweight people have tried to lose weight in the past—and failed—and gained more weight in the process, which leads to even worse self-esteem. And that's to say nothing about how being fat affects your career opportunities and even your earning potential! Fat people make less money than thin people. That is not fair, but that's how it is. Fat people are considered less attractive than thinner people, too. Society judges people that have a great lack of control over themselves and their vices. Sleep plays a tremendous role in your eating habits the next day.

LACK OF SLEEP MAKES YOU SICK

Cancer. Is there any more terrifying word? Sure, you feel crappy when you don't sleep well, but it's way more dangerous than that. When you sleep fewer than six hours a night, you have a 50 percent higher risk of developing colon cancer. And if you're a woman, consider that normally you have a 12.4 percent risk of developing breast cancer in your lifetime—if you sleep well. When you don't get enough sleep, or you don't get the quality of sleep your body needs, your risk of getting breast cancer—including the aggressive types that are more likely to kill you—is higher than that already high 1 in 8 chance.

Let's look at why. Your immune system produces B cells and T cells. These cells, called lymphocytes, identify possible attackers in your body. They're like the security screeners at the airport who identify terrorists—cells that might cause cancer and other diseases—and prevent them from getting on a plane. Phagocytes, which are white blood cells, and NK, or natural killer, cells are the police officers who arrest those terrorist cells (think cancer) and get rid of them—in this case by ingesting and eliminating them.

You may already know that your body produces melatonin, a hormone that makes you feel sleepy and helps you stay asleep. Normally your melatonin levels climb during the evening, stay high and then drop during early morning hours. Melatonin is linked with the production of T and B cells; when you are short on melatonin, you don't produce as many of these essential defenders, which means potentially harmful cells may slip through your defenses.

> " YOU GET SICK
> BECAUSE YOU CAN'T SLEEP,
> **YOU CAN'T SLEEP
> BECAUSE YOU'RE SICK** "

Lack of sleep also upsets the balance of cytokines, other substances produced by your immune system. Some are anticancer; others tend to stimulate the growth of cancer cells. Our bodies always strive for balance, or homeostasis, but when that delicate ratio of pro- and anticancer cytokines gets upset in procancer's favor, you're more likely to develop cancer. It's that simple—and that terrifying.

Lack of shut-eye makes you more likely to suffer from autoimmune disorders such as lupus, fibromyalgia, chronic fatigue, multiple sclerosis and rheumatoid arthritis. Those T cells and B cells "recognize" threats where there are none and attack your body's normal, healthy cells, causing immune disorders. It gets worse. Once you have an autoimmune disorder, that interferes with the quality of your sleep. It becomes a lose-lose scenario: you get sick because you can't sleep, you can't sleep because you're sick and you get sicker because you can't sleep.

People with chronic diseases face a constant struggle with energy levels—fatigue is the hallmark of every autoimmune disorder—not to mention the dozens of other side effects and the higher risk of death than someone who's healthy. As a result, you miss work; you're unable to spend quality time with your friends, partner and family; and you get caught up in an endless cycle of crappy sleep and feeling crappy all day long. It's a sentence I wouldn't wish on anyone, yet more than 50 million Americans deal with those side effects every day—and most probably don't realize that poor sleep may be a contributing factor.

LACK OF SLEEP MAKES YOU CRAZY

Can't sleep? Then you're likely to be depressed. At least 1 in 10 Americans deals with chronic insomnia, which is tightly linked with depression. The cost of depression in this country alone totals a staggering $34 billion in lost productivity and medical treatment, but that factor doesn't even touch the real cost of depression. As you saw in the previous chapter, depression is more than a disease. It's a soul-killing condition that many people struggle with for years, never suspecting that at least part of the cause is their inability to sleep.

If you're depressed, not only are you likely to have a less than happy existence, but you're also likely to die prematurely—regardless of your overall health—than someone who isn't. Research has found that depression is linked with inflammation, which ups your risk of developing cardiovascular disease and other conditions. And you're more likely to commit suicide; according to the National Alliance on Mental Illness, over 15 percent of clinically depressed people kill themselves. Research published in the *Journal of the American Medical Association* finds that a whopping 40 percent of people with insomnia also have a psychiatric disorder, including 15–20 percent who suffer from depression. Missing several hours of sleep just one night causes you to feel angrier, sadder, more stressed and more mentally exhausted than normal. Night after night of poor sleep can push you beyond your limits.

So what's going on? Your body produces serotonin, a neurotransmitter, in your brain and your GI tract. Serotonin plays a role in stabilizing mood, memory, learning, sexual desire and function, appetite, and sleep regulation, and it's primarily produced during deep non-REM (NREM) sleep. Interrupted sleep, or lack of sleep, means that your serotonin levels drop, affecting your mood and making you likely to experience anxiety, depression, seasonal affective disorder and obsessive-compulsive disorder.

Another factor? The loss of REM sleep. During REM sleep, your brain categorizes and stores important memories. A lack of REM sleep affects your ability to learn and remember things, but it's more significant than that. When you dream, your brain works things out. It deals with the anxieties, worries and pressures of daily life—everything from whether you'll keep your job in this economy to how you'll pay your bills to whether your husband might be falling out of love with you to where you left your iPhone. It's like a nightly therapy session.

Interrupt it—or don't get enough of it—and you don't have the insights you need to handle your life the next day. Your brain didn't have a chance to work things out the night before, so you walk around with distracting emotional baggage and worries the next day, and you're unable to embrace the new day you've been given.

LACK OF SLEEP MAKES YOU UGLY

And, yeah, when you don't sleep well, you not only feel like crap—you look like crap, too. Forget the glowing skin of someone who's well-rested. Short yourself on sleep and you'll see the results in the mirror—and so will those around you.

You already know that your body produces more cortisol when you don't sleep. Well, excess cortisol is bad for your skin—it can damage the collagen that keeps your skin looking smooth, young and wrinkle-free. If you haven't slept well—especially night after night—you'll look 10 years older, with wrinkles, bags and under-eye circles as evidence. Human growth hormone, which you learned about in the previous chapter, is released during deep NREM sleep, and helps keep your skin from thinning. Thin skin = wrinkles, and nobody wants them!

By now you should want nothing more than to get to sleep, and fast, but it's not that easy. You need a sleep reset—a way to determine what factors are keeping you from getting the sleep you need, and to set the stage for enough quality sleep. The first change you'll notice will be more energy, but your overall health, mood and even your looks will markedly improve as well!

DANGEROUS SLEEP DRUGS

There are 60 million prescriptions filled for sleep aids each year, and about 1 in 10 Americans has taken prescription sleep meds. Pharmaceutical solutions for insomnia almost always backfire. They might knock you out initially, but they often disrupt rest by blunting sleep cycles and your body's production of sleep-related hormones. Stirring or awakening from deep or dream sleep is common in people who take sleep meds, weakening the immune system, clouding brain functions and creating chaotic moods.

Eventually, the brain receptors will stop responding to sleep meds and you'll experience rebound sleep loss, setting off a vicious cycle of more fatigue, lost sex drive, insomnia and weight gain. Quality of life worsens and life span is potentially shortened. Recent research revealed startling links between common prescription sleep drugs and premature death and cancer—risk for early death was five times greater in people who take sleeping pills and risk for cancer was 35 percent higher. Just 18 pills a year could put you in this high risk group.

It's tempting to turn to a pill to help you sleep—and in our culture we do have a pill-popping mentality. Take a drug and your problem disappears. But it's more effective—and much safer—to uncover and address the causes of your sleep problems, rather than try to simply smother the symptoms. Let's take a closer look at the dangers and drawbacks of these drugs.

SIDE EFFECTS OF PRESCRIPTION SLEEP AIDS

Listen to any drug commercials for treating insomnia and you may be amazed by the side effects they list—and that's just the beginning. Common side effects of these prescription drugs include:

- ✖ Headaches
- ✖ Constipation
- ✖ Dry mouth
- ✖ Trouble concentrating/ brain fog
- ✖ Muscle aches
- ✖ Dizziness
- ✖ Unsteadiness
- ✖ "Rebound" insomnia
- ✖ Daytime sleepiness

Benzodiazepines and nonbenzodiazepines such as Ambien, the most common prescription sleep aids, are called "sedative hypnotics." They act by slowing down the nervous system. In addition to causing dependence, they can cause more serious side effects, including:

- ✖ Severe allergic reactions
- ✖ Memory lapses/problems
- ✖ Facial swelling
- ✖ Sleep-related behaviors such as sleepwalking and sleep-driving, which you are unable to recall the next day
- ✖ Sleep-eating, where you eat without remembering it the next day
- ✖ Unexplained weight gain (from sleep-eating)

These drugs also suppress REM sleep, where you work out your anxieties and fears. So you may "sleep," but you're not getting those nightly therapy sessions that are essential for positive mood the next day. Is it worth it? Of course not.

Think that taking an over-the-counter (OTC) sleep aid is safer? Well, they have their own side effects. OTC sleeping medications contain antihistamines, which are usually taken to treat cold symptoms and allergies. Antihistamines can cause the following symptoms:

- ✖ Moderate to severe drowsiness
- ✖ Blurred vision
- ✖ Clumsy or off-balance feelings
- ✖ Constipation/ urinary retention
- ✖ Dry mouth/throat
- ✖ Dizziness
- ✖ Forgetfulness

Taking sleep aids has other serious consequences as well. Many drugs become habit-forming, and you may become dependent on them. If you're used to taking them and you don't take them, your sleep problems become even worse. Even if you don't become dependent on the drug, you can develop a tolerance to the medication, which means you have to take more of the same drug to derive the same effects—and that often means you have more side effects as well. Discontinuing the drug too quickly can lead to withdrawal symptoms, such as insomnia and anxiety. On the whole, I think sleeping medications are bad news, not only for the quality of your sleep but for the quality of your life as well.

Now you know how critical sleep is, not only to your health, but also to your emotional well-being, your ability to be successful and your overall attractiveness. Don't be worried about the dangers of sleeping poorly or not enough—realize that with my plan, you'll reset your sleep habits and find that you're healthier, happier and look better, too!

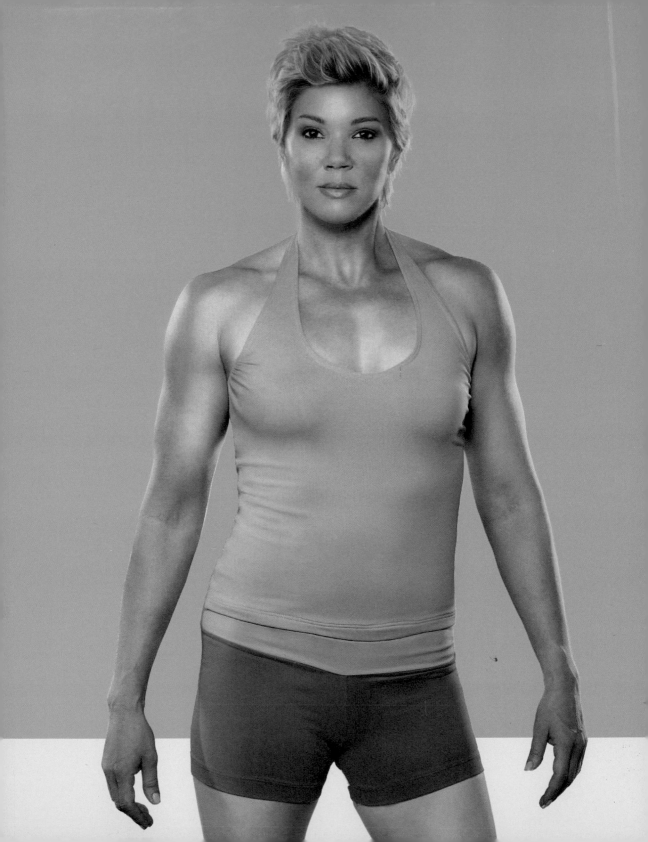

PART TWO

TRANS-
FORM
YOURSELF
FROM
BURNOUT TO
BURN BRIGHT

" IF YOU BOUGHT
THIS BOOK, IT IS BECAUSE
YOU WANT TO
**LOOK AND FEEL
AMAZING** "

CHAPTER FOUR

THE TOTAL PACK -AGE:

CELL & GLAND RECOVERY

We have discussed how turning to coffee, energy drinks, alcohol, sugar and pills to recover lost energy and to boost mood are making matters worse. You're certainly not alone in your pursuit of coping mechanisms. As I've noted before, for a time even I started relying on quick fixes that affected my health and energy in a negative way. I have prescribed every diet and exercise program offered here for myself first and then for my personal clients, fine-tuning and perfecting them, finally, to give to you.

THE THREE PHASES

I created this program with three distinct phases. In Phase 1, you'll consume a primarily vegan diet to intensively detox sickly cells in just seven days. Only whole foods that are easily broken down for digestion will be consumed, freeing up cells to get maximum absorption of nutrients. During Phase 1, you'll eat fresh vegetables and fruits rich in oxygen, phytonutrients and antioxidants to flush out toxins and repair mitochondria. The surge of nutrients from increased consumption of "out of the box" foods—powerful, plant-based foods found only in the produce section—will create an energized environment in the body, accelerating tissue repair and boosting circulation for faster cell cleansing. Cell-strengthening proteins will be from beans and plant sources alone.

In Phase 2, you'll focus on restoring hormonal harmony. When this is achieved, the body orchestrates energy, calm and confidence with ease. In Phase 2, you'll consume foods and spices that balance insulin levels and hormones, creating maximum internal stability. The foods will promote steady energy and quality sleep by normalizing adrenal and thyroid functions, and create cleaner metabolic functions by accelerating glucose turnover and regulating insulin response.

Now that you've gotten the first two phases of the program completed, you'll switch gears to focus on adding muscle. You'll move up to 1,800 calories per day of lean proteins and fat-burning, muscle-building carbs. To maximize muscle and create a lean and toned shape, you must consume foods that feed muscle. Phase 3 focuses on the dynamic duo of muscle boosting: amino acids and glycogen.

PHASE 1: DETOX

In Phase 1, you'll remove negative crutches while adding foods and exercises specifically designed to powerfully revive your cells. You will see and feel an immediate difference. In the first seven days—Phase 1—the venti lattes, processed snacks and too frequent alcohol consumption will be replaced with very specific foods that contain very specific nutrients for cell and gland repair. Your cravings for "negatives" will dissipate and give way to cravings for the foods in this program. Remember, your cells are literally starving for nutrients and your body and brain will reward you with positivity on a molecular level. Weight gain, poor skin, anxiety and exhaustion will dissipate and give way to daytime energy and nighttime balance.

Let's first address total cell repair, a complete rebuilding of the energy engines that dictate how you look and feel. Healthy cells keep your energy up and your weight down. When you restore these, you will be beautiful from the inside out!

If you bought this book, it is because you want to look and feel amazing. My program will rejuvenate all your cells, but our specific focus will be on healing the cells or parts of the cells most responsible for looking beautiful, gaining energy and preventing sickness. Let's take a closer look at how we will rejuvenate your cells.

STRONG BATTERIES = **High Energy**

MITOCHONDRIAL REGENERATORS

These foods help boost your cells' ability to produce energy, or ATP, which stands for adenosine triphosphate. ATP is the fuel that powers your body's cells.

You now know that your energy level is a direct result of the energy production happening in your cells. Let's take a look at what happens when your mitochondria are functioning optimally, like an engine that burns clean. You wake up feeling rested and energized, ready to tackle your day. You feel bright and poised to engage. You have energy to spare—enough to hit the gym after the office for a challenging workout, start your own business or run your family with finesse.

Better yet, you avoid that crash after dinner—instead of lying lifelessly on your couch, you feel motivated to spend time with your family or head out to meet friends. And as the day winds down, you feel tired but not exhausted. That's what healthy mitochondria do for you!

My plan includes foods chosen specifically for their ability to regenerate the mitochondria and produce clean energy. These foods have been proven to make the batteries of your cells run at full power.

Mitochondrial regenerators include:

COQ10	ALPHA-LIPOIC ACID	MANGANESE
Peanuts	Spinach	Raspberries
Sesame seeds	Broccoli	Wheat germ
Pistachios	Collard greens	Hazelnuts
Broccoli		Pine nuts
Cauliflower		Pecans
Oranges		Pumpkin seeds

COQ10	ALPHA-LIPOIC ACID	MANGANESE
Strawberries		Sesame seeds
		Sunflower seeds
		Brown rice
		Quinoa

STRONG MEMBRANE = **Balanced Mood**

MEMBRANE STRENGTHENERS

You learned in chapter 1 that healthy cellular membranes are closely associated with mental health. Your cell's membrane is the skin of the cell, but its role is much more important than simply enclosing the cell. Nutrients pass through the membrane and cellular wastes are expelled through it. Without a healthy membrane, your cells cannot receive the essential nutrients they need and garbage builds up, making them toxic.

Even more important, though, is the membrane's role in intercellular communication. Within your membrane are the neurotransmitter transporters, the signaling messages that communicate with nearby cells. Healthy membranes carry the correct messages to the correct cells. But weak or damaged membranes can't do that. Their transporters malfunction and cellular communication goes haywire; that's akin to when a text message gets sent to the wrong phone.

As a critical example, consider when the neurotransmitter serotonin isn't correctly communicated between the cells. On the big-picture level, this means your mood isn't stable. You may feel anxious one moment, depressed the next. You're irritable or snappish without knowing why, or fly off the handle at even the most minor of setbacks. Or you may feel like you've always got a case of the "blues," even though you have plenty of wonderful things in your life! Moods gone haywire are a sign of malfunctioning membranes, as is a negative outlook or loss of joy that you just can't seem to shake.

Just as some foods help power up your mitochondria, specific foods also help maintain healthy cellular membranes, which are essential for positive mood and reduce your risk of anxiety, depression and related disorders. During this detox, you're already eliminating most saturated fats and all trans-fatty acids, both of which can damage cell membranes.

This program includes membrane strengtheners like the following:

OMEGA-3 FATS	CHOLINE	VITAMIN E
Walnuts	Peanuts	Spinach
Chia seeds	Potatoes	Almonds
Cauliflower	Cauliflower	Hazelnuts
Mung beans	Lentils	Sunflower seeds
Whole oats		Avocados
Sesame seeds		Olive oil
Flaxseeds		Broccoli
		Squash

NUCLEUS PROTECTORS

As I just mentioned, your cellular membrane is essential for stable, positive mood and an optimistic outlook. In addition to your outer cell membrane, the nucleus of your cells contains its own nuclear membrane, designed to help protect its DNA. So when you protect the nucleus, you also protect your DNA.

Each of your cell's DNA is like a tiny user's manual that tells each of your body's cells exactly what to do.

STRONG NUCLEUS = Healthy DNA

When your DNA gets damaged, however, your cells go a little crazy, so to speak, and malfunction. That leads to all kinds of diseases and autoimmune disorders.

Healthy DNA is the key to overall health, not only for you, but also for your children and grandchildren as well. As I pointed out earlier, when your DNA is damaged, it not only increases your risk of developing all kinds of diseases, including killers such as cancer, but you also pass along subpar DNA to your children.

But let's focus on you first. When your DNA is damaged, or mutated, that means the cell gets scrambled instructions. DNA gets damaged all the time; that's part of living in today's world and being exposed to all kinds of toxins and chemicals. If your DNA repair process is working at 100 percent capacity, or close, any cells that go "rogue" can quickly be brought back into line. If your body is able to repair the damaged DNA, you can turn off the "switch" that is making those cells turn cancerous and get them back to following the user's manual. Here's how:

+ STEP 1: Protect the nucleus and DNA with a healthy cell membrane.

+ STEP 2: Make the DNA less susceptible to damage.

+ STEP 3: Repair that DNA before it goes rogue.

And how do you repair that DNA? By eating the specific foods I have chosen to protect and repair your DNA.

Nucleus/DNA protectors include:

VITAMIN A	BETA-CAROTENE	FOLATE
Carrots	Green leafy vegetables	Sunflower seeds
Sweet potatoes	Cantaloupe	Spinach
Dark leafy greens	Melons	Turnip greens
Butternut squash	Carrots	Collards
Dried apricots	Sweet potatoes	Mung beans
Cantaloupe		Pinto beans
		Chickpeas
		Asparagus
		Peanuts

By now you should be getting very excited that your cells are going to heal, getting you on track to a healthier and happier you. My plan will increase cell power, giving you energy; strengthen cell walls, enhancing your mood; and repair damaged DNA, keeping you out of the doctor's office and off prescription meds. Everything in life improves when you become the captain of your own ship. Sickness and sadness no longer rule your life when you take control of your own health through your new lifestyle.

BEAUTY *OR* THE BEAST

HEALTHY DERMIS CELLS = Plump Collagen = Youthful Appearance

We've been talking about the types of foods that will protect and power up the three essential cellular components. Now let's take a closer look at how boosting cell function through diet and exercise will not only make you healthier but make you more attractive as well.

While you see only the outer layer of skin, the epidermis, it's the second layer, the dermis, that makes a huge difference in your appearance. (The third layer, the hypodermis, is where your body stores fat.) Your dermis is the layer of skin cells that contains collagen, a protein that—along with another protein called keratin—makes your skin smooth, strong, elastic and resilient.

As babies, children and young adults, our bodies produce plenty of collagen, which makes for smooth, flawless skin and silky, shiny hair. As we get older, however, our bodies produce less collagen, and our skin becomes weaker, less elastic and more prone to wrinkles and lines. We get "laugh lines" around our eyes and mouth. Our neck starts to sag as collagen production decreases, and even if we're fit, we notice that the skin on our torso and limbs isn't as "tight" as it once was. If you've never had cellulite, this loss of elasticity may mean that you suddenly notice lumps and bulges you never saw before.

I can spot someone whose skin cells are sick a mile away; they're dull in both energy and appearance. Lack of collagen doesn't just lead to wrinkles—it causes rusty joints, too. Collagen makes up about 30 percent of your body's proteins and is also used to form connective tissues, such as ligaments, tendons and skin. You want your collagen cells to be lush, hydrated and fat; that's better for flexibility and elasticity in your joints and critical to creating youthful, taut skin. When referring to collagen, "skinny" carries a very negative connotation.

As you age, collagen grows thin and deflated due to declining estrogen and testosterone levels, which inhibit the cells responsible for producing collagen and elastin. But it's not just growing older that is hurting your collagen production.

Ugly daily habits include:

* ✖ Consistently eating sugar
* ✖ Consistently drinking alcohol
* ✖ Drinking less than two liters of water daily
* ✖ Smoking of any kind

Okay, so now you're saying, "Jackie, thanks for making life a complete bummer!" Don't worry—you can reintroduce sugar and alcohol in moderation, once you've reset your system.

Failing to hydrate will make your collagen cells weak and less plump. And sugar from food and alcohol introduces harmful, protein-damaging molecules that dry out collagen cells. When these proteins are thin and thirsty, you get wrinkles, saggy skin, cellulite and painful joints. In our youth-obsessed culture, people will do anything to reverse the signs of aging. What always amazes me are the drastic measures that we will go to in order to look younger when the solution is so much simpler: do things daily that plump up collagen, making those collagen cells fuller and healthier. This detox will jump-start your body's collagen production and within a week, you'll look younger, healthier and more attractive!

Yes, time is working against you. But we know that there are certain foods that help boost collagen production, whether you're a 20-something, a 40-something or beyond!

"YOU CAN'T STOP GETTING OLDER, BUT YOU CAN MAINTAIN A VITAL, YOUTHFUL APPEARANCE"

To plump up your collagen and improve your dermis cells for a beauty boost, you'll be eating foods high in the following:

LYSINE	HYALURONIC ACID	CATECHINS/ ANTHOCYANIDINS	VITAMIN C
Beans	Potatoes	Green tea	Red/green hot chili peppers
Peas	Sweet potatoes	Blackberries	Bell peppers
Lentils	Bananas	Raspberries	Guava
Peanuts	Beans	Cherries	Kale
Chickpeas		Apples	Mustard greens
Pinto beans		Pears	Broccoli
Pistachios		Fava beans	Brussels sprouts
Sunflower seeds		Red cabbage	Kiwifruit
Pecans			Papaya

You can't stop getting older, but you can maintain a vital, youthful appearance. When I go to the movies, I look closely at the actors I think are aging gracefully, then I go home and find information about their lifestyle. Every single time I've done this, the actresses and actors who are wrinkled yet beautiful have a very healthy lifestyle and it shows in their skin. People with plenty of collagen may develop a few lines as they get older, but their skin has a suppleness and glow of someone half their age.

Because of their skin's overall health, they look a decade or more younger than their calendar age. The quantity of their years is not reflected in the quality of their skin! This detox program will give your collagen in particular and your skin in general the boost they need to start turning back the clock on your appearance.

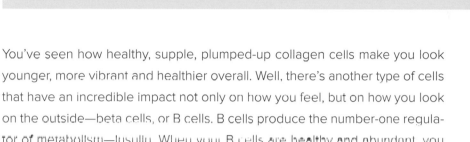

HEALTHY B CELLS
= Balanced Insulin = Healthy Weight

You've seen how healthy, supple, plumped-up collagen cells make you look younger, more vibrant and healthier overall. Well, there's another type of cells that have an incredible impact not only on how you feel, but on how you look on the outside—beta cells, or B cells. B cells produce the number-one regulator of metabolism—insulin. When your B cells are healthy and abundant, you go from a fat-storing to a fat-burning machine. B cells regulate metabolism by secreting insulin after you eat, in response to glucose, or blood sugar. Think of insulin as the key that unlocks the door to your cells, and lets the glucose into the cells to feed them. Without insulin present, your cells will turn away the glucose and your metabolism crawls instead of runs. This means weight gain or a stubborn inability to lose weight.

A healthy or "fattened" B cell ensures steady energy, regulates cravings, eliminates compulsive eating, triggers good moods and feelings of calm, and promotes weight loss. Powerful B cells also boost immune function and reduce your risk of developing insulin resistance or type 2 diabetes. Certain nutrients improve the health and vitality of B cells, including fructose, a natural sugar found in fruits. The only type of fructose you should consume comes from whole fruits, not artificial sources. For example, eating products with high-fructose corn syrup can interfere with normal B-cell function and cause weight gain and diabetes.

To boost and bolster your B cells, you will eat the following:

BIOTIN	ZINC	IRON	SELENIUM
Swiss chard	Steel-cut oats	Spinach	Brazil nuts
Carrots	Asparagus	Collards	Whole-grain bread
Almonds	Peas	Kale	Sunflower seeds
Walnuts	Pumpkin seeds	Prunes	Sesame seeds
Strawberries	Sesame seeds	Raisins	Crimini mushrooms
Raspberries		Beans	Brown rice
Onions		Lentils	
Cauliflower		Chickpeas	
		Artichokes	

Healthy B cells act as the key to the door of your cells to get blood glucose where it needs to be—inside your cells. My detox plan will eliminate the unhealthy fats that harm B-cell function and power your B cells with the specific foods they need to get your metabolism revved and keep your energy levels steady. As a bonus, your increased B-cell function will help you shed extra pounds—by week's end you'll already notice that you're slimmer, with energy to burn.

IMMUNE SYSTEM RESET

Your B cells work in conjunction with T cells, which help identify toxins and spur your immune system to respond to them. T cells can malfunction, though, and when this happens, your immune system attacks your body's own healthy cells, causing autoimmune disorders. More than 50 million people now suffer from autoimmune disorders, including what I call the "big four":

✖ Fibromyalgia

✖ Lupus

✖ Chronic fatigue syndrome

✖ Psoriasis

It may surprise you that my mother and I suffer from two disorders on this list. My mother has fibromyalgia, which she treats with the exercises and diet that I have given her. I came down with a case of mononucleosis when I was 27, which gave me Epstein-Barr syndrome, which gave me chronic fatigue syndrome. I remember being exhausted by 11:00 in the morning and then struggling through the day as best as I could.

Not until I radically changed my diet did I effectively treat my symptoms. I haven't felt those symptoms for years and even though the virus is still in my blood, I have amazing energy every day. These chronic disorders seriously compromise quality of life in those who suffer from them as well as their friends, family and colleagues. Millions of people with autoimmune disorders struggle to work and get very depressed as a result of their symptoms. I'm here to tell you that your diet can either cause terrible symptoms—or eliminate them.

We will reset your body's immune function by avoiding trans-fatty acids—these accelerate inflammation, which is linked to autoimmune disease—as well as incorporating healing foods. This detox plan also resets your body's immune system so that it functions the way it's designed to. Now, for example, when precancer cells form, as they do in all of us, your healthy cells will rush in to eliminate them and prevent them from harming you.

You can change the course of disease and instead of suffering on a surgeon's table, live the last chapters of life with vibrancy and health. Your health starts with your cells, but your immune system plays an important secondary role in combating and eliminating the many poisons that make their way into your body. This program will help *all* your cells—including B cells and T cells that are integral to the body's immune system—function at close to or at 100 percent.

Foods that reboot your immune system include:

BETA-CAROTENE	LYCOPENE	LUTEIN
Green leafy vegetables	Tomatoes	Kale
Cantaloupe	Guava	Spinach
Melons	Watermelon	Broccoli
Carrots	Red cabbage	Corn
Sweet potatoes	Grapefruit	Brussels sprouts
	Asparagus	Oranges
		Tangerines
		Tomatoes
		Carrots
		Papayas
		Melons

COMBAT STARVING CELLS

Another benefit of this detox is that it combats two common problems most of us deal with every day without realizing it—"hidden hunger" and malabsorption.

Hidden hunger is the nutrient deprivation that comes from a lack of whole-food consumption or a heavily processed diet. Hidden hunger leads to weight gain and chronically feeling and looking unhealthy due to anorexic cells. The consumption of factory-farmed meats deepens deficiencies in vitamins B, C, D and K, and essential minerals such as zinc, magnesium and calcium. These deficits damage the cell, creating fatigue, moodiness and a sluggish metabolism.

These nutrient-deprived cells are starving—and a starving cell will either break itself down too much or too little, either of which can result in cancer, autoimmune diseases, inflammatory diseases or viral infections.

In the short run, when people are consistently undernourished, they become just like a light stuck on dim—they possess no brightness or energetic thrill for life. Symptoms include:

✖ Irritability

✖ Fatigue

✖ Depression

✖ Inability to think with clarity

✖ Hair loss, thin skin and dark under-eye circles

✖ Frequent sickness

✖ Reduced sex drive and fertility problems

✖ Weight gain

Foods causing hidden hunger include:

✖ Processed and deli meats, and nonorganic dairy products

✖ Snack bars

✖ Packaged snacks

✖ Canned foods

✖ Boxed foods

✖ Fried foods

✖ Candy

✖ Salty, processed snack foods

✖ Nonorganic produce

If this sounds a lot like the way you eat, don't worry; our cell detox is going to nourish those starving cells from the inside out. When you detox your cells and then feed them what they need, you'll help prevent hidden hunger.

MALABSORPTION

Even when you do eat healthy foods, you may not get the nutrients you need from them. Malabsorption occurs when your body is unable to digest certain vitamins, proteins or carbohydrates. It causes symptoms including the following:

✖ Bloating

✖ Cramping

✖ Gas

✖ Diarrhea

✖ Nausea

✖ Muscle wasting

It's bad that the average American does not eat enough nutrients. Worse is the fact that even when you try to increase nutrient consumption, your out-of-whack cells can't properly absorb them.

What do you do when that "apple a day" may deliver only 30 percent of its nutrients? Take a multivitamin, right? Well, in all likelihood, that vitamin is not being absorbed and used by the body in amounts that will keep you healthy and energetic. Most Americans are deficient in three key vitamins and minerals: magnesium, a mineral essential to energy production; vitamin B_{12}, critical for boosting cell energy; and vitamin D, which plays an important role in mood and energy.

Most people with malabsorption don't know they have it, but are often plagued by symptoms such as weakness and fatigue. The idea of a hard workout is repellent to them, as their bodies are just not equipped to handle it.

Blame this inability to absorb vitamins on:

- ✖ Processed diets
- ✖ Sugar and artificial sweeteners
- ✖ Prescription medications

The foods in this program will not only give your cells meganourishment but they will also help the cell absorb almost all the nutrients that foods can bring. Many of you have heard the statement "Eat to live, don't live to eat," meaning eat healthy foods to function, not only the comfort foods that give you pleasure. You will see that soon you will "live to eat" these cell-nourishing foods, and that your body and brain will crave them, which makes your healthy lifestyle a lot easier to manage.

MEDS AND MALABSORPTION

We're a pill-popping nation. We fill 310 million prescriptions for antibiotics each year and 30 million Americans take anti-inflammatory medications *every day*! Another 30 million of us regularly take sleeping pills, and about 10 percent of adults take an antidepressant.

The continual use of drugs has made our intestines unable to absorb the nutrients our cells so desperately need. If you take any of these drugs regularly you may be experiencing malabsorption:

- Antibiotics
- Oral contraceptives (birth control pills)
- Estrogen replacement therapy
- Anticonvulsants
- Diabetes medications
- Antihypertensive meds (to lower blood pressure)
- Anti-inflammatories (ibuprofen, aspirin)
- Anti-ulcer and heartburn drugs (H2 blockers, such as Prilosec, Nexium)
- Cholesterol-lowering drugs
- Beta-blockers
- Phenothiazines (for mental disorders)
- Tricyclic antidepressants
- Benzodiazepines (for anxiety and insomnia)

Malabsorption can also lead to the same cellular responses as hidden hunger; cells can either break themselves down in an attempt to get the necessary nutrients, or become

> suicidal if their nucleus is damaged beyond repair. But while malabsorption is common, it's relatively easy to fix by making a positive change in your diet.

One more thing. *When* you eat is just as important as *what* you eat. During Phase 1, and thereafter, you will be eating breakfast, a snack, lunch, a snack and dinner with no more than three hours between consumption. (In Phase 3, you'll add a postworkout snack, too.) Keep your daily meal intake close to this:

7:00 a.m.	Breakfast
10:00 a.m.	Snack
1:00 p.m.	Lunch
4:00 p.m.	Snack
7:00 p.m.	Dinner

Well, I hope you are feeling that your cells are about to be awakened. I want you to think of this detox as giving a gift to yourself and your cells. Your body is a beautiful machine and wants to work perfectly. You are well on your way to feeling and looking great!

PREBIOTIC POWER

Prebiotics are parts of food that cannot be digested but that stimulate the bacteria in the digestive tract. Prebiotics also improve immune function, since your digestive system is an important part of your immune system.

I've included the following powerful prebiotics in my program:

- Bananas
- Honey
- Garlic
- Onions
- Apples
- Oats

> " WHEN YOU HAVE WORN-OUT ADRENALS, YOU CRAVE FOOD AND DRINKS THAT CAUSE A QUICK ENERGY SURGE **ONLY FURTHER BREAKING YOUR ADRENALS DOWN** "

PHASE 2: BALANCE

THE ADRENAL CLEANSE

It's not only your cells that need detoxifying; you will be cleansing your glands during the 21-day detox as well. As you read in chapter 2, your lifestyle choices are likely causing adrenal fatigue. If your glands were healthy, simply drinking a glass of cold water or eating an apple would be a healthy and natural pick-me-up. But when you have worn-out adrenals, you crave food and drinks that cause a quick energy surge only further breaking your adrenals down.

When your adrenals are burned out, you notice it from the moment you wake up. You're groggy when you first get up, relying on caffeine to jump-start your day. Your mood is erratic—you may feel depressed, anxious, listless or irritable with no real reason. And your energy levels, already low, continue to plummet throughout the day until around dinnertime when you get an unexpected energy surge. Unfortunately, this interferes with your body's normal circadian rhythms and makes it difficult for you to sleep, which restarts the cycle all over again.

As you read in chapter 2, you're exposed to adrenal toxins as a result of living a developed-world lifestyle. However, food is a very powerful medicine, and my detox plan will also cleanse your adrenal glands of toxins, the first step to normal adrenal function. On this plan, you won't be consuming sugar, caffeine, alcohol, energy drinks, fast food or packaged crap, which will give your adrenals a break.

One of the keys to adrenal function is the types of foods you eat, and when. On this plan, you'll eat protein-carb pairs, which have a "time-release" effect on blood sugar. This stabilizes blood sugar—chaotic blood sugar strains hormone production in the adrenals and causes wild mood swings as well. On the first seven days of my plan, you'll eat vegan protein-carb pairs such as these:

+ Garbanzo beans and veggie salad
+ Oatmeal and mixed berries
+ Avocado sandwich with veggies and sprouts
+ Carrots and hummus
+ Apple and walnuts
+ Celery and nut butter

Another key to eating to cleanse and reboot your adrenals is to eat small meals throughout the day. Most people eat in a crescendo throughout the day: we skimp on or skip breakfast, relying on coffee to keep us going; grab some fast food that's laden with salt and fat for lunch; and then overeat at dinner and snack well into the evening. That erratic dietary pattern wreaks havoc on adrenal function.

Instead, on my detox plan you'll be eating small, regular meals that will stabilize the adrenals' hormonal production. The foods that detox and reset your cells will do the same for your adrenal glands. The whole grains; dark leafy greens; nuts, seeds and legumes; richly colored fruits and vegetables; and healthy fats will clean up your adrenals and help them balance your body functions.

One big solution is that now you will be eating the right kind of breakfast every morning—even if you're not hungry. To combat adrenal fatigue, you must consume the right nutrients that keep insulin and cortisol levels balanced. This will keep your adrenals from stressing out.

As you read in Phase 1, eating the right foods at the right time of day is very important. You will continue eating breakfast, a snack, lunch, a snack and dinner with no more than three hours between meals and snacks.

And, of course, the quality of the food you eat is critical. My plan includes foods essential for adrenal support, including non–animal-sourced protein (think legumes) to help reboot adrenal function. Heart-healthy oils will help increase healthy cholesterol, from which the adrenals manufacture hormones.

In Phase 2, I'm building on Phase 1, and have selected specific foods that will cleanse your adrenal glands, including the following:

VITAMIN B$_5$	CHROMIUM	VITAMIN B$_{12}$
Brown rice	Broccoli	Chili peppers
Whole grains	Garlic	Almonds
Mushrooms	Apples	Wheat bran
	Bananas	Sesame seeds
		Sun-dried tomatoes

Eating the foods included on this detox plan, and eating throughout the day will cleanse your adrenal glands—and help them power up to produce the right amounts of hormones throughout the day, resulting in steadier energy, a more positive mood and weight loss as well.

THYROID REHAB

Finally, in Phase 2 and thereafter, we'll be rebalancing the thyroid. Many people suffer from either an over- or underactive thyroid. But when your thyroid is balanced, you wake up feeling rested and calm. Everyday stressors roll off your back, and you're able to focus both at work and at home. Your mind is clear, ideas come to you easily and you're able to keep up with your to-do list without struggling. Your digestive system functions normally, and you have no trouble maintaining a healthy weight. You can tell your thyroid is optimal by simply looking in the mirror—your hair is shiny and strong, and your skin is supple and strong. When your thyroid is balanced, and producing the optimal amount of hormones, you feel good both inside and out.

However, whether your thyroid tends to be overactive or underactive, the end game is misery! Instead of taking medication to try to adjust your thyroid function, we'll do it through healthy, nutritious, specially chosen foods.

Phase 2 includes foods that will rest your thyroid and help it function optimally. You already know that on my detox plan you'll be eating healthy fats such as omega-3s. (After the first seven days, we'll add other powerful animal sources of omega-3 fats.) While some people rely on omega-3 supplements to make sure that they're consuming enough, our bodies appear to absorb these essential fats more completely when they come from foods, not supplements.

These specific foods will help rehab an overactive or underactive thyroid:

VITAMIN B$_6$	VITAMIN C	TYROSINE
Brown rice	Red/green hot chili peppers	Almonds
Whole grains	Bell peppers	Avocados
Pistachios	Guava	Pumpkin seeds
Garlic	Kale	Sesame seeds
Sunflower seeds	Mustard greens	Lima beans
Sesame seeds	Broccoli	Bananas
Hazelnuts	Cauliflower	
	Brussels sprouts	
	Kiwifruit	
	Papaya	

Healthy Oil Choices

I'm a fan of extra-virgin olive oil, and have used it in the recipes throughout Phase 2 and Phase 3. "Extra-virgin" oil is the least processed olive oil (produced by pressing the olives themselves); it's the least acidic of any olive oil, and has the freshest flavor, which makes it a great choice for salad dressings and topping lean protein. However, if you like, you can try coconut oil in the dressing recipes instead. While coconut oil is a saturated fat, it consists of medium-chain fatty acids, not long-chain fatty acids found in animal-produced saturated fats. That difference makes coconut oil easier for your body to absorb, and its unique makeup appears to help improve metabolism and optimize thyroid function. Coconut oil is also being studied for its apparent role in reducing the risk of heart disease, cancer and other diseases.

The choice is yours. Both oils (and flaxseed oil, found in the smoothies) are heart healthy choices.

TOP 10 TO DEFEND

Here are the top 10 foods that power up your glands and boost cell production:

- Broccoli
- Red and green peppers
- Raspberries
- Kale
- Chickpeas (including hummus)
- Sesame or sunflower seeds
- Almonds
- Lentils
- Steel-cut oats/ whole grains
- Carrots

FOOD INTOLERANCES

I hear a lot of clients *saying* that they have food intolerances, when they may actually be the victims of poor diets—namely, diets that contain too many processed foods full of additives and too few sources of enzymes the body needs to digest that food! A food intolerance occurs when your body is unable to digest the food in question. People with lactose intolerance, for example, often lack enough of the enzymes that break down lactose, and suffer from gas, bloating, upset stomach and diarrhea when they consume it.

These symptoms typically come from overeating processed dairy or bread products or a nutrient-deficient diet that lacks specific enzymes you need to digest these foods completely. While people are usually told to avoid foods that cause reactions, consuming foods that contain specific enzymes can help them overcome food sensitivities.

There are now hundreds of gluten-free options on store shelves, but you should know that only about 1 percent of people have celiac disease and are unable to digest gluten found in many grains. People with celiac disease are unable to break down and digest other essential nutrients; this causes digestive problems and can lead to more serious conditions such as anemia and osteoporosis. Many more of us have a sensitivity or intolerance to gluten (or lactose or other foods), which causes minor but annoying digestive problems. So if eating bread makes you feel bloated or pasta sends you to the potty, you're likely to have a less serious sensitivity than true celiac disease.

I've helped hundreds of clients overcome food sensitivities by having them eliminate processed food from their diet and focus on fruits, vegetables, whole grains and organic sources of protein. Eating this way helped rebuild their intestinal flora so that they were able to add the foods they were formerly sensitive to with no ill effects! This 21-Day Detox program will help you do the same.

PHASE 3: LEAN

Once you've detoxed your body's cells and reset your glands, it's time to add muscle. You'll be eating more calories than you did in Phase 1 and Phase 2; your body needs more energy during this phase of my program to provide your muscles with the nutrients needed to repair the damage done and build new, stronger muscle tissue. You'll be eating enough to build that muscle and to have plenty of energy during the rest of the day, too. The Lean Food Plan is high in protein, to build muscle tissue, and both simple and complex carbohydrates, to nourish that tissue.

Muscle runs on glycogen, the form in which carbohydrates are stored for long-term energy use. Stocked glycogen stores will provide all-day, rock star energy levels. And amino acids will give you the top-quality materials needed to create dense, calorie-burning muscle tissue. Your glycogen stores will respond best to fruits (fructose) and starchy vegetables, which break down easily to maltose and can quickly be converted to glycogen.

You'll consume whole grains for maximum fiber, which will power digestion and accelerate glycogen storage. For amino acids, lean proteins are the optimal sources, especially those highest in essential amino acids, which are not produced by the body and must be provided through diet. You should eat these clean animal sources of protein three times a day. A selection of optimal glycogen and amino acid sources includes the following:

FRUCTOSE	FIBER AND STARCH	WHOLE GRAINS	CASEIN	ANIMAL PROTEIN SOURCES
Apples	Broccoli	Quinoa	Greek yogurt	Lean roast beef
Raspberries	Beets	Brown rice	Whey protein	Chicken and turkey (without skin)
Pineapples	Sweet potatoes	Whole-grain pasta/bread	Low-fat cottage cheese	Fish
Avocados	New potatoes	Nut butters		Shellfish
	Corn	Lentils		
	Squash			
	Peas			

NATURAL DETOX SUPPLEMENTS

■ **CURCUMIN:** Curcumin is the active ingredient in turmeric. Along with the spice cumin, curcumin gives some Indian and Thai curries their mustard color. Taken as a supplement, curcumin is a powerful antioxidant that has anti-inflammatory, antimicrobial and anticarcinogenic effects. This means it helps your body crush cancer cells and ward off inflammatory diseases. Science shows it's particularly effective at improving gastrointestinal health because much of it gets absorbed directly into GI cells.

■ **CRANBERRY EXTRACT:** Take cranberry extract to accelerate the detoxifying effects of my exercise and eating plan. Cranberry extract is rich in proanthocyanidins, which prevent bacteria and toxins from sticking to cells in the body—if they can't stick, you won't get sick. The antioxidants found in cranberries will also work to cleanse the lymphatic system and the kidneys, which will increase energy and give you radiant skin.

"BEING BEAUTIFUL IS NOT ABOUT BEING SKINNY. **IT IS ABOUT LOOKING HEALTHY**"

CHAPTER FIVE

STRONG IS THE NEW SKINNY: THE WORK -OUTS

In the previous chapter, you learned about what to eat to detox your cells and glands. In this chapter, you'll learn about foods and exercises that will make you your most powerful, giving you the edge in life to do anything you put your mind to!

I have studied the effects of muscle for over two decades and have not only transformed my own genetically challenged body, but have guided thousands through a complete transformation as well. I love muscle and you will, too, when you learn all the amazing things it does for you!

Muscle is active in repairing every function of the body, from skin to organs to DNA. It is a critical key to energy, metabolism and mood. Having more muscle will drastically change body and brain chemistry, giving you the confidence and energy to have a more passionate life. I call it the attraction amplifier, boosting energy, accelerating weight loss, reducing disease and sickness, relieving stress and simply making you look and feel a lot hotter. I'm a fan!

A person lacking in muscle will burn fewer calories; build up more metabolic waste, which can lead to inflammation; have poorer circulation, leading to low energy, cloudy thinking and a sickly skin tone; and, perhaps worst of all, have the appearance of a slouch (this includes skinny people, too!).

In fact, muscle mass has been shown in research to be the biggest predictor of longevity, recovery from illness and overall health.

If muscle came in a bottle, everyone would buy it. But it's not that easy; while you have some muscle already, you have to strength-train to maintain it. Most of us are undermuscled and overfat. Even if we're at a "normal" weight, our bodies lack the muscle to keep our metabolism and energy levels high.

VANITY VERSUS VITALITY

It's time to redefine beauty to yourself. Being beautiful is not about being skinny. It is about looking healthy. Researchers have found that people rate attractiveness by "signals of quality"—and having muscle tone suggests grade A health. We want to see ourselves partnering or procreating with those who will boost our own brand. I believe that a toned and healthy body actually gives you "star power."

Star power is the charisma that you exude when you feel a strong inner confidence about personal qualities and appearance. I did not have this until I really took hold of my life, and learned how to set goals and achieve them. At 21, I started training my body to be beautiful and strong. As my body changed, my personality became much more confident. That confidence led to many personal achievements and created a cascade of opportunity. When I tell you that strength training changed my life, I really mean it.

We judge people on attractiveness using different standards, but, in general, women find men who have a V-shaped torso with broad shoulders and a narrower waist physically appealing. Men generally like women with a low waist-to-hip ratio, a number that typically indicates a healthy percentage of body fat, and muscle helps keep that percentage at appealing levels.

A higher proportion of muscle does more than make you look sleek and strong. It means you have better blood flow, and your skin is likely to look radiant and glowing, another factor associated with physical attractiveness. Research proves that just 12 weeks of regular weight training significantly improves body image in both men and women. That means your body language is confident and assured, and people are attracted to confidence in both men and women.

This undeniable energy and charisma can be found by anyone. It is not defined by your looks; it is defined by how you carry yourself. A toned, healthy body gives you added strength and confidence that will attract others.

THE WORKOUTS

My workout plan includes three phases: Phase 1: Prime Routine; Phase 2: Burn Routine; and Phase 3: Mean Routine. Let's take a look at each phase and its purpose.

PHASE 1 WORKOUT: **PRIME ROUTINE**

GOAL: Engage Your Brain

LENGTH: 7 days

You now know how to eat to cleanse your body's cells and fine-tune your glands. You'll also help reset your body's hormonal and cellular health by performing the gentle but challenging workout this week. The overriding goal of the prime workout is to "prime" your muscles for work. You'll work out six days this week, but in a slow, controlled fashion. For example, you'll do four sets of squats, 10 repetitions each, while focusing on perfect form.

By doing my specifically selected moves, you'll start to create the mind-muscle connection that helps you build muscle more quickly, and makes your workouts engaging for both body and mind. In the second stage of the program, you'll focus on strengthening your heart, and during the third stage, you'll focus on creating more lean muscle.

CREATE THE MIND-MUSCLE CONNECTION

Tell me, do you hate working out? It's okay if you say yes. That just tells me that you haven't made the mind-muscle connection yet. Here are three things holding you back:

✖ You don't know how to work out efficiently.

✖   You overdo cardio and skimp on weight training.

✖   You view weight training as manual labor and resist it at all costs.

I guarantee that I will teach you the most effective exercises done in the most effective combinations that you can easily remember and take with you any-where. Cardio work alone does not change your body type; it is actually the slowest way to drop weight. By the end of this program, you will have changed your mind-set. Exercise is not something you *have* to do; it is something that you will *want* to do because you will see and feel all the amazing things that come with it.

Workouts are a way to connect with all parts of yourself and go into a meditative state when your mind is clear and great bursts of creativity occur. All the ideas that have made me successful and happy in the past 10 years were conceived when I was in this state of mind-body connection.

Remember, the body is greatly affected by our thoughts. Science is beginning to understand the degree to which the nature of thoughts and emotions actually determine your health and strength. When you know how to mentally connect to your muscles during workouts, you can increase growth by 30 percent. Here are a few tips while training:

✚   Go into your workout with a positive attitude, as if you were going on a new adventure.

✚   Listen to upbeat and fast music. Go to www.JackieWarner.com for playlists.

✚   Focus on each muscle that you are working as you work it.

✚   Visualize yourself as strong and athletic.

✚   Chase the burn. Even if you're feeling fatigued, focus on performing each rep with the intention of muscle burn and growth.

Your goal during the first week is to practice the mind-muscle connection that will help you get more from your cardio and strength workouts in the coming weeks. You'll follow the Phase 1 diet described in chapter 7 and consume about 1,300–1,550 calories a day.

PHASE 2 WORKOUT: **BURN ROUTINE**

GOAL: Burn Maximum Calories

LENGTH: 7 days

Phase 1 was about connecting your mind with your muscles. Now we're going to move into Phase 2, where you'll strengthen your heart *and* your muscles.

These workouts include multijoint exercises, which use more muscle groups and burn more calories overall. Your heart will be challenged to force blood to your lower and upper extremities, which will make your heart strong and keep you burning calories for several hours postworkout.

Multijoint or compound movements involve lifting using more than one joint, therefore impacting many muscle groups at one time. More muscle tissue is worked, burning more calories. Your nervous system and stabilizer muscles will be more stimulated. Multijoint exercise puts a good stress on the heart because it is forced to pump more blood to multiple muscle groups. And studies show that testosterone levels rise most rapidly when you train using heavy weights and target multiple muscle groups with multijoint exercises. This means you're setting the stage to add the lean, metabolically active muscle that you need.

If fat loss is your main goal, then multijoint, whole-body exercises should be the base of your program. Squats, dead lifts and presses are all considered multijoint but for maximum burn we will be combining two at a time, such as performing a squat and a bicep curl simultaneously.

HEART POWER

Challenging your heart muscle by exercising at a high intensity has numerous benefits for your body. Simply put, the heart is a muscle—the most important muscle of your body. While any cardiovascular exercise is good for you, the harder you (safely) work your heart, the more benefits you get. You will be greatly strengthening your heart through these multijoint exercises and you'll be able to harness that power—and that means you will have more stamina, a more positive outlook and the ability to tackle your day and still have energy left over for the things you're passionate about.

This workout will do more than increase the power of your heart; however, by keeping your heart rate elevated for short periods, you'll train not only your heart but also your entire cardiovascular system. When you circuit-train, you perform different moves one after the other, with little to no rest. So you might do squats, then push-ups and then lunges with no rest. The idea is that, while you're using different muscle groups, you're always working at a relatively high intensity. This keeps your heart rate up, burning calories and strengthening your heart and lungs.

You may have heard of high-intensity interval training, or HIIT. This kind of training has been proven to boost your body's aerobic fitness, burn fat and raise metabolism, and my workouts are HIIT, which studies show boosts your fitness level faster than any other type of workout. As a result of this workout, your lungs and the rest of your cardiovascular system work more efficiently and carry more oxygen and nutrients to your cells. Cardio exercise also boosts the number of mitochondria in your cells, and helps repair damaged mitochondria as well. It increases insulin sensitivity, which helps stabilize blood sugar levels, and encourages healthy gland function.

The Tread Is Dead

Forget about spending hours on the treadmill if you want to lose weight and keep it off. Steady-state cardio exercise won't do nearly as much to help you lose weight and get healthy as doing interval workouts and strength training. The latest thinking is all about building muscle through strength training, and doing short bursts of high-intensity exercise. Well, my plan does both—and because your heart rate increases and stays up during your workouts, you get the benefits of an aerobic workout—without being bored on the treadmill.

Circuit training, the way we do it in this program, also has a significant impact on your mood, both in the short and long term. Aerobic exercise has been shown in some studies to be as effective as medication for treating depression and anxiety, and even short bursts of high-intensity exercise boost mood.

During this week's workout, you'll follow the Phase 2 diet described in chapter 8, and consume about 1,600 calories a day.

PHASE 3 WORKOUT: **MEAN ROUTINE**

GOAL: *Add Lean Muscle*

LENGTH: *7 days*

After the first two phases, it's time to up the ante with Phase 3: Mean Routine. Think of the last seven-day phase as *power*. Powerful amino-acid-containing foods, coupled with powerful movements, will quickly change the way you look and feel. Women, do not be afraid that you will "bulk up." The foods and structure of the exercises, together with your body's lower testosterone levels, will keep you from looking like a linebacker, I promise. You will just become the best, hottest version of yourself—you will find your inner athlete.

I'm a fighter. If you tell me no or that something cannot be done, I work and fight to prove the opposite. My workouts are consistently in the "mean" zone. This means you will get more done in a half hour than most people do all week. Your body and brain want to live in this zone. The result of a mean workout is a day that you will burn bright with passion and intensity. Imagine what this will mean for your career and/or your family.

I'll be honest. This workout isn't easy! But a mean workout is worth three or four of the so-so workouts you're probably used to doing. With a mean workout, you'll perform up to 10 repetitions and experience muscle failure, meaning that you've exhausted your muscle's capabilities. The harder you work that muscle, the more results you'll get from your workout.

I've designed this workout with power in mind. Not only will you take your muscles to failure—which means they'll rebuild stronger, leaner and more metabolically active than ever before—you'll also use "ladder" training, where you increase the number of reps you do for a certain exercise and then decrease it again (think of climbing up and then descending a ladder). You'll feel the ultimate burn on the last few reps, and recruit more of these fast-twitch muscles that jack up your metabolism and help you stay young and vital.

THE FAT AND FATIGUE DEFENDER

Muscle tissue will accelerate metabolism by turning over calories three times faster than fat—one pound of muscle burns 50 calories every day. Plus, once muscle is activated, it continues burning calories for several hours. Muscle tissue also releases AMP-activated protein kinase (AMPK), an enzyme that directly improves energy metabolism by turning on fat-burning and improving beta cell function for better insulin regulation. As your body provides your muscle cells with the nutrients they need to grow, your metabolism stays elevated—so even when you're sitting around, you're burning more calories than you would have if you hadn't lifted weights earlier that day.

The same tissue that will give you shapely shoulders and sexy legs will also boost energy. Muscle tissue holds more mitochondria than any other tissue, which is why with more muscle will come great increases in energy. Like anything else in life, if you don't use it, you lose it. But muscles adapt quickly and in just one day can change your metabolism and energy levels. Clients who tone up report off-the-charts energy levels. They look amazing, too.

TIMING IS EVERYTHING

As you saw when we talked about Phase 1: Detox, it's also important to feed your muscles at the right time. Yes, good nutrition is essential for healthy, vibrant cells, but nutrient timing—eating the right things at the right time—will help you build muscle faster and keep you consistently burning fat throughout the day.

You already know that your body needs carbohydrates, protein and fat as part of your diet. Your muscles specifically require glucose, or sugar, and amino acids, which make up protein, to stay powered up. For this reason we will change breakfast into preworkout and postworkout meals. Before working out, you will eat protein/carbs and after working out you will eat protein/carbs and good fat.

This is the combination that best fuels your muscles, which are starving for the right balance of protein and carbs and healthy fat postworkout. An example of a preworkout meal is a cup of oatmeal with a cup of berries mixed in. This will give you both quick and sustained energy for the workout itself. A perfect postworkout meal would be two eggs with citrus fruit and a piece of whole-grain toast. Your pre- and postworkout meals are the most important of the day because that is when your muscles are going to be hungriest and searching for energy to grow.

When you strength-train as with my circuit plan, your muscles deplete their store of glycogen and the fibers break down. If you don't feed your muscle cells what they need, your body will actually eat the muscles for energy, making you weak in body and mind. The 30- to 45-minute "window" postworkout is when your muscles are the most receptive to glucose and rebuilding. Taking in carbohydrates and protein together will replenish your body's glycogen stores and help your body repair the damage to muscle cells that strength training produces.

Eating immediately after working out raises insulin levels that have fallen during exercise. It also suppresses the production of cortisol and other hormones, and spurs the muscle and liver to replace and store glycogen. This slows down the muscular breakdown and speeds up repair and recovery. The Lean Food Plan is higher in protein with specific carbs that will only help you build lean muscle and burn excess fat.

During this week's workout, you'll follow the Phase 3 diet described in chapter 9 and consume about 1,800 calories a day.

So here's what your eating plan might look like in Phase 3 if you work out first thing in the morning. Your normal mealtimes will stay the same; the only difference in the schedule is your postworkout snack.

7:00 a.m.	Breakfast
8:00 a.m.	Postworkout Snack
10:00 a.m.	Snack
1:00 p.m.	Lunch
4:00 p.m.	Snack
7:00 p.m.	Dinner

MORE MUSCLE, LESS DISEASE

The more muscle you have, the better equipped your body is to fight off infection and diseases both minor and severe. Your muscle cells produce and store glutamine, an amino acid, and immune cells need glutamine to function. When you're fighting off an illness, your muscle cells release glutamine into your bloodstream to power your immune cells; the more glutamine you have stored, the better equipped you are to fight off infections. This is why doctors are now starting to focus more on helping older patients build more muscle—not only does it improve their mobility and reduce their chances of injury, but it also reduces their risk of succumbing to disease.

Recent research has also revealed that contracted muscles secrete small proteins called myokines, which create an anti-inflammatory environment that is also antidisease. By suppressing inflammation, myokines prevent disease pathways from forming in the brain and body. By contracting muscles, you set up a body environment that:

✛ Fights bone loss

✛ Fights weak joints and breakdowns in connective tissue

✛ Fights all heart disorders

✛ Fights insulin spikes and slow metabolism

✛ Fights cancer

✛ Fights autoimmune disorders

✛ Fights anxiety

Both men and women start to lose muscle in their 30s. My plan will not only prevent you from losing muscle—it will also help you create new muscle that will improve your overall health.

Muscle doesn't just make you look better on the outside; it improves your body's health on the inside as well. We know that weight training helps prevent the following conditions:

+ **TYPE 2 DIABETES.** When you add muscle, you improve your body's ability to manage your blood sugar, which helps moderate the symptoms of diabetes and can prevent you from developing it.

+ **OSTEOPOROSIS.** You may not be worried right now about developing osteoporosis, but this disease, caused by brittle or thin bones, affects millions of women and men, and can cause disability. Build strong muscles and you'll also build strong bones and increase your bone density, which makes you less likely to break a bone now and to develop osteoporosis in the future.

+ **LOWER BACK PAIN.** Four out of five people suffer from back pain in their lives, and it is the second leading cause of lost worktime. Just as frightening, back pain is the third most common reason to have surgery and the fifth most common reason to be hospitalized. And here's the thing: when your back hurts, it means you're often unable to do anything. Chronic back pain is also linked with depression—no surprise there.

+ **OSTEOARTHRITIS.** While this is the most common form of arthritis, weight training helps reduce its symptoms by strengthening joints and connective tissue. As muscles around joints get stronger, they protect those joints from injury.

+ **DEPRESSION.** I've already talked about how depression is at near-epidemic levels. Building muscle decreases depression, improves self-esteem and boosts self-confidence.

- **HEART DISEASE.** It's the number-one killer of Americans, but weight training helps reduce your body's overall fat, which in turn reduces your risk of cardiovascular disease.

- **AUTOIMMUNE DISEASE.** Moderate weight training can help reduce the achy, stiff joints associated with autoimmune diseases such as rheumatoid arthritis, lupus and fibromyalgia. When you weight-train, it's not only your muscles that get larger and stronger. Your cartilage, tendons and ligaments also become thicker and stronger; this connective tissue strength reduces painful autoimmune disease symptoms and makes you more impervious to common injuries.

- **ANXIETY.** While cardiovascular exercise appears to be more effective in treating depression, strength training is just as effective at managing symptoms of anxiety.

But strength training does more than ward off disease. Strength training also helps galvanize motor units that were previously inactive; as your central nervous system senses you need "more power," nerve signals prod other motor units to get in the game. Each motor unit is made up of a nerve that connects to muscle tissue; when these motor units fire, your muscles work. Think of your motor units as football players lounging on the sideline until the coach points at them and says, "Hey, you! Get out there!" Then they jump into the action.

MORE MOTOR UNITS = More Power = More Mitochondria = More Energy

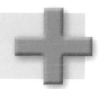

It's truly a win-win situation!

FREE WEIGHTS OVER FACE-LIFTS

Research into longevity has revealed that muscle tissue is your ultimate defense against aging. As we age, skin and tissues may lose volume, taking on a thin, saggy look. To regain fullness and a youthful skin tone, you'll rebuild skeletal muscle, the tissue type that rests just beneath the skin all over your face and body. When you use resistance training to build muscle, you send a surge of oxygen, nutrients and water to these cells, which creates a volumizing effect.

By training muscle, you also increase collagen cells, and promote greater production of growth hormone (nicknamed the "youth hormone" for a reason). Both work to repair and strengthen tissue connections, giving you a tight, toned appearance.

MOTHER NATURE'S NATURAL RELAXANT

Forget about anti-anxiety meds! Give your muscles a good workout and your hormone and neurotransmitter receptors will become more responsive, increasing the effectiveness of the body's calming chemicals. More muscle also balances the autonomic nervous system (ANS), which regulates reaction (as part of the fight-or-flight response) and relaxation. A balanced ANS weakens the effects of stress by stabilizing your blood pressure and heart rate, leaving you calm and cool even in the midst of an overburdened life.

Must-Have Muscle Supplement

Branched-chain amino acids (BCAAs) are a group of amino acids that should be on your go-to list of supplements. They are typically made up of leucine, isoleucine, valine and other essential amino acids. Your immune and muscle cells will gobble up BCAAs and use them to replenish and repair tissues, speed up metabolism and generate new cells. You'll feel more energized, too, since BCAAs delay tryptophan delivery to the brain, pushing "pause" on fatigue. This means you can work out more intensely, and that you'll have more energy throughout the day as well.

You'll get better sleep, too, with more muscle tone—consistent training increases production of the sleep hormone melatonin, which means you'll get to dreamland faster and avoid interrupted sleep cycles.

As you'll see in the next chapter, people who strength-train regularly have better sleep quality than those who don't. That means they fall asleep more quickly and sleep longer than people who don't train, possibly because strength training increases the production of human growth hormone, or HGH, which is linked with better sleep.

In fact, a survey conducted by the National Sleep Foundation and published in 2013 found that people who exercise have better-quality sleep than those who don't exercise. The higher the level of exercise, the bigger the impact—people who exercise vigorously sleep the best of all and rarely, if ever, have symptoms of insomnia. So let that be a motivator for you if you ever feel like skipping a workout—exercise not only creates more energy but sets the stage for high-quality sleep, which in turn begets more energy, and the cycle continues.

In chapter 4, you learned about the way you'll eat to detox your cells, reset your body's glands, and add lean muscle to your body. In this chapter, you learned why adding lean muscle is the single best thing you can do for overall health, vitality and beauty. In the next chapter, we'll add the final component—getting the sleep you need for optimal physical and emotional health.

"THE MOST IMPORTANT KEY TO GETTING QUALITY SLEEP IS THE REGULATION OF HORMONES THAT PRODUCE CALMNESS AND ENERGY"

CHAPTER SIX

EXTREME SLEEP MAKE-OVER:

HORMONAL RESET

The most important key to getting quality sleep is the regulation of hormones that produce calmness and energy. In an unhealthy, out-of-whack system, hormones transmit confused messages, causing energy hormones to fire at night and calming hormones to be withheld. When these hormones are rebalanced, your mood will improve, a calm, relaxed state will come easily, and you'll suddenly feel as though you've tapped into a steady, incredible source of energy. In this chapter, I'll share a strategic plan for recovering and rebalancing hormones critical to sleep and better well-being: cortisol, oxytocin, prolactin and progesterone.

These four hormones play different roles in the body, but in general cortisol and prolactin are sleep-killers and oxytocin and progesterone are sleep-promoters.

TOO MUCH CORTISOL = Bad Sleep
TOO MUCH PROLACTIN = Bad Sleep

ENOUGH OXYTOCIN = Quality Sleep
ENOUGH PROGESTERONE = Quality Sleep

It's as simple as that. The sleep mystery is easily solvable once we control these hormones. So let's look at the two hormones we want to suppress for sleep, and the two we want to promote for better, beautifying sleep.

THE CORTISOL COCKTAIL

Cortisol is commonly known as the "stress hormone" and has gotten a bad rap in the weight-loss industry. Yes, too much cortisol is linked to belly fat, but cortisol is a strong *energy hormone*, and it should be balanced, not banished. When the right amount of cortisol is produced, you'll feel alert and grounded and even be protected from the effects of stress throughout the day. The key is to regulate cortisol so that it turns on for energy during the day, when you need it, and turns down for calm at night.

We balance cortisol by enhancing brain health. Specifically, the pituitary gland, located in the brain, will send signals that are translated by the adrenals. The key is to consume foods that give the pituitary the right instructions while keeping the adrenals functioning properly so that cortisol is regulated. In chapter 2, you learned that adrenal fatigue affects about four out of five of us, and that one of its major symptoms is chronic fatigue. The right amount of cortisol powers you up to cope with stressors; too much overloads your body's adrenal system and leads to a constant feeling of exhaustion, although you may notice a surge of energy in the early evening. That surge isn't a "second wind" because you had no energy earlier in the day! Instead, it's a sign that your adrenals are malfunctioning and churning out more cortisol when they should be shutting down for the day.

Normally your cortisol levels gradually rise in the early morning hours (this helps give you the get-up-and-go to get out of bed) and then continue to climb, with some fluctuations, through the day. In the early evening, they start to drop to prepare your body to relax and set the stage for sleep.

To help reset your cortisol levels and produce the perfect cortisol cocktail, we need more 1) monounsaturated fats, 2) magnesium, 3) selenium, and 4) vitamin C. Monounsaturated fats have a proven link to balanced hormonal output from the hypothalamic-pituitary-adrenal axis (HPA axis), which is where cortisol and other important hormones originate. When the HPA axis is operating smoothly, daytime energy is high, anxiety is low and sleep is solid. You need magnesium to regulate cortisol production, and to relax muscles, setting you up for better sleep. When levels of the potent antioxidant vitamin C are low, cortisol goes up and immune health and collagen synthesis go down. New research also shows that vitamin C is associated with good sleep; people who consume more vitamin C sleep more (on average, seven to eight hours a night) than those who don't.

Thanks to the cell-boosting foods you started consuming in Phase 1, and the Phase 1 workout, you may have already noticed that you're sleeping better. You read in chapter 4 why I chose certain foods for Phase 1 and Phase 2 (recall that in Phase 3, you follow the same plan, but add a healthy postworkout snack and extra protein). Well, I chose the foods for Phase 2 with quality sleep in mind. The diet during Phase 2 is designed to reset these four hormones, including cortisol. You'll eat foods containing:

MONOUNSATURATED FATS	MAGNESIUM	SELENIUM	VITAMIN C
Olive oil	Black beans	Brazil nuts	Tomatoes
Peanut oil	Pumpkin seeds	Oysters	Red bell peppers
Nut butters	Swiss chard	Nuts	Watermelons
Olives	Halibut	Seeds	Apricots
Avocados		Lobster	Oranges
		Tuna	
		Sunflower seeds	
		Lean beef	
		Lean pork	
		Dark meat/ chicken/turkey	

> **"** THANKS TO THE CELL-BOOSTING FOODS YOU STARTED CONSUMING IN PHASE 1, AND THE PHASE 1 WORKOUT, YOU MAY HAVE ALREADY NOTICED THAT **YOU'RE SLEEPING BETTER "**

OXYTOCIN: THE LOVE HORMONE

Oxytocin has been called the love hormone, and it's what helps creates a bond between mother and newborn child. Oxytocin also helps us feel connected and close to lovers, friends and family members. The more oxytocin we produce, the calmer and happier we can feel, and the better we're able to buffer the effects of too much cortisol. This makes for better, more restful sleep. To increase oxytocin and balance cortisol, make time for personal connections; phone calls and instant messaging can lower cortisol and promote oxytocin, but in-person experiences, especially those that include hugs or affection, go further in creating a sense of calm.

The best way to boost oxytocin production is to incorporate more activities that produce it. Try these:

+ Have sex. Sex doesn't just feel good; it ramps up your oxytocin as well. Kissing, touching, snuggling, foreplay and actual sex all increase oxytocin, and an orgasm produces levels two to three times higher than normal.

+ Touch someone. Sex may be one of the best ways to boost oxytocin, but simply touching someone else increases it as well. Physical contact is essential for high levels of oxytocin. If you're not having sex, get a massage; you'll get similar benefits. And don't be stingy with hugs or hand-holding.

+ Love your pet. Petting, playing or holding an animal is a proven stress-reducer and oxytocin-producer.

✚ Shift your mind-set. Your thoughts have a powerful impact on your mood and outlook and can affect hormone production as well. Focusing on happy memories, thinking about people you love, or simply fantasizing about positive things can boost oxytocin.

✚ Laugh. Get together with a friend who always cracks you up or watch your favorite comedy. With YouTube, you have millions of videos at your fingers to make you laugh, which increases oxytocin.

✚ Treat yourself. Instead of grabbing a glass of wine at the end of a long day, choose a hot bath. Listen to your favorite music. Burn candles and create an ambience that is pleasing. The activities that you find relaxing and pleasurable will turn on the production of oxytocin as well.

There are some dietary ways to help boost oxytocin, too. Consuming healthy fats will cause your small intestine to produce a hormone called cholecystokinin, or CCK. This hormone triggers the release of oxytocin, which then causes a feeling of satiety. Choosing foods that have positive connections for you—say, hearty oatmeal that your mom used to make for you on cold winter mornings—will also produce more oxytocin. You'll include in your diet foods that contain healthy fats, such as the following:

HEALTHY-FAT-CONTAINING FOODS

✚ Avocado	✚ Flaxseed oil
✚ Extra-virgin olive oil	✚ Nut butters
✚ Coconut oil	✚ Walnuts

PROLACTIN

Prolactin is a hormone produced by the pituitary gland. High prolactin is far more common than low levels of prolactin, so we'll focus on regulating rather than raising levels of this important hormone. When prolactin is balanced, it has a positive effect on fertility, sex drive and sleep quality. To instigate proper timing of prolactin release, we'll work on boosting dopamine and regulating the neuropeptide galanin.

Dopamine is a neurotransmitter that is essential for a healthy, high-functioning metabolism. It also works in the brain's "reward center." When you eat food you like or perform an activity you enjoy, dopamine is released in the brain. (Drugs such as cocaine and meth have a similar effect, which is why they're so addictive.) You can see that the production of dopamine parallels that of oxytocin; activities that produce the one are likely to produce the other and vice versa.

PLEASURABLE ACTIVITIES = More Dopamine

You need high dopamine to restrain prolactin production, but with too much galanin, dopamine is hard to come by. Galanin is involved in a variety of functions, including regulating mood, sleep and appetite, but too much of it interferes with dopamine production. So we've got to balance both for the right amount of prolactin production. The plan during Phase 2 (and from here on out) includes foods with tyrosine, B_6, betaine and zinc, which may help increase production of dopamine.

You'll also consume foods that contain B-complex vitamins and vitamin E, both of which help suppress elevated levels of prolactin. Eat foods like these:

TYROSINE	VITAMIN B_6	BETAINE	ZINC
Wheat germ	Bananas	Beets	Oysters
Avocados	Potatoes	Whole grains	Crab
Almonds	Pistachios	Spinach	Peanuts
Eggs	Sunflower seeds	Broccoli	Pumpkin seeds
Poultry	Sesame seeds	Shellfish	
Cottage cheese	Wild-caught salmon		
Lima beans	Yellow-fin tuna		

PROGESTERONE: MORE THAN A SEX HORMONE

You've seen how your diet in this week of the program will reset your cortisol balance and how the proper diet, along with engaging in activities you enjoy, will also help boost oxytocin. Now let's talk about the role progesterone plays in sleep. Progesterone is a sex hormone that works in conjunction with estrogen and is known for its importance in fertility and healthy pregnancy.

However, it's critical for a variety of functions besides reproduction. Progesterone helps build bone mass. It increases insulin sensitivity, which helps maintain stable blood sugar levels, and lowers your risk of developing diabetes. It also improves and stabilizes mood, helps the body break down fat and increases energy production. This hormone is also sexy—it boosts libido and sex drive—which makes you more likely to increase your level of oxytocin, too! (See how these two good hormones are linked?) And, just as important, progesterone is associated with quality sleep.

> " TOO-LOW PROGESTERONE CAN CAUSE WEIGHT GAIN, ANXIETY, POOR SLEEP, MOOD SWINGS AND INTERRUPTED SLEEP. **PROGESTERONE IS A KNOWN PROMOTER OF SLEEP** "

Men naturally have lower levels of progesterone than women, but women typically start to notice a decrease in progesterone in their 30s. Too-low progesterone can cause weight gain, anxiety, poor sleep, mood swings and interrupted sleep. Progesterone is a known promoter of sleep—during pregnancy, levels of this hormone go up and contribute to increased sleepiness. We want production to be turned up at night and turned down during the day. This creates better sleep, solid daytime energy, stronger immune health and increased use of fat for fuel.

To produce more progesterone, you'll eat more foods with plant sterols, naturally occurring substances in plants that lower bad cholesterol by blocking its absorption. You'll also increase consumption of inflammation-lowering foods, such as those that contain vitamin C, vitamin E and omega-3 fats, and avoid xenohormones as much as possible. Xenohormones are "strange" or "alien" substances that disrupt your natural production of estrogen, testosterone and progesterone. They're a type of endocrine disruptor, which you learned about in chapter 2, that interfere with normal thyroid function. Sources of xenohormones include:

✖ Nonorganically farmed livestock (cattle, pork, poultry and sheep) that have been fed estrogenic drugs to help them gain weight more quickly. (This is another compelling reason to choose organic, or what I call "clean," meat whenever possible.)

✖ Artificially created sex hormones used in oral contraceptives and hormone replacement drugs. (This applies even if you don't take these drugs, as they get into the water supply and you can be exposed to them without even knowing it.)

✖ Many pesticides, fungicides and herbicides.

✖ Bisphenol A. You already know from chapter 2 how widespread BPA exposure is; in your body, its estrogenic effects increase your risk of certain cancers, including breast and prostate.

The less exposure you have to xenohormones and other endocrine disruptors, the better. I suggest you eat only organic foods, particularly meats. Avoid drinking water from plastic bottles; instead, use an aluminum bottle, which is better for you and the environment.

You'll also consume plant sterols, which reduce "bad" cholesterol without impacting "good," or HDL, cholesterol needed for progesterone production. And since high C-reactive protein (CRP) levels are linked to low progesterone, lowering inflammation is important to regaining hormonal balance. (The liver produces CRP in response to inflammation.) You'll also eat foods to help boost progesterone, including the following:

PLANT STEROLS	VITAMIN C	VITAMIN E	OMEGA-3 FATS
Whole grains	Red/green hot chili peppers	Spinach	Flaxseeds
Rice bran	Bell peppers	Almonds	Walnuts
Wheat germ	Guava	Hazelnuts	Salmon
Oat bran	Kale	Sunflower seeds	Sardines
Brown rice	Mustard greens	Avocados	Grass-fed beef
Peas	Broccoli	Olive oil	Halibut
Beans	Cauliflower	Broccoli	Scallops
Lentils	Brussels sprouts	Squash	Shrimp
Peanuts	Kiwifruit		
Almonds	Papayas		
Walnuts			
Sunflower seeds			
Pumpkin seeds			

QUALITY SLEEP = Quantity Energy

Ultimately, cortisol, prolactin, oxytocin and progesterone should sync up with your body clock to promote sleep at night and wakefulness during the day. Whether regulating these hormones improves sleep or improving sleep promotes better hormone regulation is a bit of a "chicken or egg" debate. My plan will help you attack fatigue and feeling low from both sides to ensure optimized energy levels. The next step is to create an environment and lifestyle that is conducive to good sleep.

I always wondered why I slept so wonderfully and deeply in hotels but tossed and turned at home. What I discovered was that my bedroom environment was completely counterintuitive to restful sleep. I made the following changes and now I sleep peacefully through the night.

Making these changes will help you become a super sleeper with energy to spare the next day:

+ **Set a schedule.** When you get up and go to bed at about the same time each day, your body becomes habituated to falling asleep at that "set" time. As a bonus, it's easier to get up the next morning, too! I realize that some nights—say, on the weekend—you may wind up going to bed later than you'd like. Even so, get up at the same time in the morning and you'll help ensure that you sleep well that night. You may be tired after a late night, but it's better to maintain your sleep schedule than to try to catch the Zs you didn't get.

+ **Go dark.** Many of our bedrooms are nowhere near dark—and the darker your room, the better. You should have blackout curtains that don't even let the moonlight in. Even dim light has been linked to disturbances in the hippocampus, the region of the brain linked most to moods. Also, light triggers cortisol production, which wakes us up. Your pineal gland produces melatonin, which makes you sleepy. Melatonin is turned on by the dark; light interferes with the production of melatonin. Even the LED lights on your VCR or alarm clock can produce enough light to interfere with sleep, so cover them or make sure that they don't add more light into your bedroom.

+ **Turn off, tune out.** Stop staring at your phone, or any other screen, 30 minutes before going to sleep. Ninety-five percent of Americans say they use some type of electronic device right before bed.

Research shows that the light used in smartphones, computers and TV screens is melatonin-suppressive. This means it actually delays the production of the hormone your body uses to signal "lights out." Turn off, tune out and pick up a good book right before bed instead. If you feel stressed at the idea of going to sleep without a quick check of email, make it at least a half hour before you go to bed. That will reduce the impact on melatonin production—and keep you from being stressed out over an email or text before you turn in. Keep your phone outside your bedroom and don't check it throughout the night. I know, it might sound scary to go to sleep without it at

Super Sleep Snacks

Want to sleep better? Give these power snooze snacks a try:

- **WALNUTS.** Walnuts contain tryptophan, an amino acid essential to the production of serotonin and melatonin.

- **SALMON, HALIBUT AND TUNA.** No, you may not want a piece of halibut right before bed, but a dinner that contains one of these types of fish, which are high in vitamin B$_6$, another precursor to melatonin, can help you drop off more quickly later on.

- **ALMONDS.** They're high in magnesium, which is associated with solid sleep.

- **LOW-SUGAR, WHOLE-GRAIN CEREAL AND ORGANIC MILK.** The combination of complex carbs and calcium increases tryptophan levels, and the calcium helps you relax. (So your mom was right about that glass of warm milk before bed!)

- **BANANAS.** This popular fruit contains tryptophan, which helps induce sleep.

- **ORGANIC GREEK YOGURT.** The calcium in Greek yogurt helps reduce stress and can help you relax into sleep.

arm's reach. But the fact that you know it's there is disturbing your sleep. Instead, make your bedroom your retreat for sleep (and sex), as you'll see below, and keep the electronics out of it.

+ **Exercise. Hard.** A poll conducted by the National Sleep Foundation found that vigorous exercisers rarely have sleep problems and report getting a good night's sleep most nights of the week. Even moderate and light exercisers were "significantly more likely" to report sleeping well compared to nonexercisers. And despite what you may think, recent research suggests that working out right before bed isn't likely to affect your sleep quality; a 2011 study published in the *Journal of Sleep Research* found that men and women who biked 30 minutes before going to bed slept just as soundly as those who didn't.

+ **Use your bed for sleep and sex only.** Strengthen your association with your bed and sleep by making sure that's one of the only activities you do there. Don't let your office overflow into your bedroom or turn it into an extra entertainment center. Sleep experts recommend not even putting a TV in your bedroom if you can avoid it. But if you do have a television, turn it off well before you go to sleep—and keep in mind that watching stressful or violent shows (even the news) is likely to interfere with your ability to fall asleep.

+ **Skip the nightcap.** Alcohol is a major disruptor of sleep stages. It may seem like a shortcut to sleep, but only the first 90 minutes will pass uninterrupted. After that, sleep cycles are disrupted—its sedating effects wear off, but sugar and cortisol spikes go up. If you enjoy a glass of wine at night, drink it early, ideally four to six hours before you go to bed, so it won't interfere with your sleep.

+ **Last coffee call at 2:00 p.m.** It can take the body six to eight hours to eliminate caffeine from the system. When caffeine is present, neurons in the brain fire, signaling the adrenals to produce adrenaline. This means that even if you're exhausted, adrenaline will work against the desire for sleep. Keep in mind, too, that some people are more sensitive to caffeine than others. If you have trouble sleeping, try refraining from caffeine in the afternoon to see if that makes a difference.

+ **The dog has to go.** When it's time for sleep, put pets and kids in their own beds. You may not be aware of it, but their movements while sleeping are interrupting your normal sleep stages. And every time you wake up, you interrupt your sleep cycle, forcing your body to start over before you can reach stage 4, the deepest, most restorative level of sleep.

+ **Cool off.** You'll sleep better in a cool room (between 60°F and 68°F) than one that's too warm. A cool room helps lower your body's core temperature, encouraging sleep. And interesting research has found that chronic insomniacs have higher core body temperatures at bedtime than those who sleep better.

+ **Choose a presleep snack.** Going to bed on an empty stomach may interfere with your sleep. You'll find the perfect sleep-promoting snacks on page 128.

BEYOND SLEEP: THREE SIMPLE WAYS TO GET AN EDGE

Of course, getting quality sleep and building lean muscle are only part of my program to reboot your body's cells and recapture your best "you." There are other things you can do that will make an appreciable difference in how you look, feel and live, such as these three simple ways to improve your life:

ACTIVE DAYDREAMING

In today's plugged-in world, we're constantly connected, and the result is that we're easily distracted and over-whelmed. Take five minutes every day to sit and meditate, or to simply breathe. You don't need to take a special class, wear special clothes or even designate a special place to sit.

In this time, I want you to visualize yourself as a strong and powerful being. Think specifically about the things you would like to achieve in life and imagine yourself doing them. I do this every day and the exact thing I have visualized for myself has come true. Once, I was visualizing that I was sitting with Oprah and I imagined the questions she would ask and what I would reply. Two weeks later, the *Oprah* show called and I was talking to her. I have hundreds of examples of this happening and if you put active daydreaming into practice, you will, too.

DRINK IT IN

I start my day with a cup of coffee and one liter of cold water. This has allowed me to keep my caffeine intake low as well as really speed up my metabolism. Drinking three liters of water a day speeds up your metabolism by about 33 percent. That's huge! When you drink cold water, your body burns calories to bring the water up to your body's temperature. That increases your overall metabolic rate, boosting your energy. Cold water also wakes you up and refreshes you; the contrast between the warmth of your mouth and throat and the chill of the water just feels great! Most of us walk around chronically dehydrated, and simply drinking more water staves off hunger pangs and makes it easier to eat a clean diet—without suffering!

Being dehydrated makes you tired, listless and out of it, and it ages your skin, too. I look at a glass of cold, clean water as one of the simplest and healthiest ways to lift my energy and my mood.

CREATE WHITE LIGHT

Ever been around someone who just sapped your emotional reserve, an "energy vampire"? (Or maybe you are the energy vampire.) I make it a point to energetically prepare myself when I walk into a room with others. My strong energy can either light up a room or really bring it down. You, too, have a tremendous responsibility to uplift others wherever you go. When you do, the exchange of happiness and connectivity will really boost your spirits throughout the day and make you feel content about yourself. Try to envision that you carry a brilliant white light within your chest and that is what people will see and feel before they see the superficial.

BEAUTY SLEEP

Women throughout the ages have discussed the importance of getting beauty sleep. But what does that mean? How does getting a solid night's sleep affect our looks?

THE BODY

Remember that in chapter 3 you learned that not sleeping enough—or not getting the quality sleep you need—makes you fat. People who short themselves on Zs, getting less than six hours a night, are almost eight times likelier to be overweight than those who get 7.7 hours a night. We know that sleepless nights interfere with other hormones, including leptin, an appetite suppressant. Yet it increases ghrelin, which stimulates appetite, at the same time! That means you're hungrier than you would be normally, especially for high-fat and high-carbohydrate foods.

It doesn't stop there, though. When you're rested, you're more likely to make smarter food choices and bypass the crap. Your resolve is stronger. Your energy is greater, which makes you more likely to hit the gym—or just spend time doing things other than lazing around on your couch, texting a friend to cancel because you lack the energy to get out of the house.

THE FACE

You already know that you don't look your best after a night of interrupted or poor-quality sleep. Well, the people around you can see the difference, too—a study published in the *British Medical Journal* found that people who hadn't slept well were rated as being less healthy, more tired and less attractive than those who felt well-rested!

When you've slept well, the blood flow to your skin is enhanced, and the result is healthy, glowing skin. That improved circulation also makes little lines less visible and gives your skin a lustrous glow. You look younger, happier and all-around more attractive!

GET ZS—GET SMART!

After a night of little or poor-quality sleep, your day starts off with unusually high cortisol levels. That makes it harder to concentrate and affects your decision-making ability.

When you get quality sleep, however, your hormone levels are balanced, and you're able to think more clearly, focus on demanding tasks and perform better at work and at home. With today's demanding schedules and constant multi-tasking, this is more important than ever before. Quality sleep is an essential ingredient to a successful career and to being able to reach your personal and professional goals.

GOOD SLEEP = **Positive Outlook**

Lack of sleep is closely associated with poor mental health, especially depression. Not only does a key feel-good hormone, serotonin, go down, but you feel physically drained, which causes a negative attitude. You're crankier and short with people—certainly not as inviting as when you feel good and rested.

Consistent sleep loss will cause more days with a negative attitude and really start affecting your personality and its energy force. Success and well-being are all connected to the energy you are giving and getting throughout the day.

SEVEN HOURS A DAY KEEPS THE DOCTOR AWAY

Poor sleepers are more likely to have autoimmune diseases, including fibromyalgia, lupus and chronic fatigue. This is because of sleep's critical role in immune function. Normal sleepers produce enough melatonin, the hormone that is linked with T and B cells, which helps your immune system identify and eliminate potential threats. So getting quality sleep means your immune system functions better overall. It produces enough T cells, B cells and cytokines to keep your body in balance and reduce your risk of getting sick, whether it's catching a cold or developing cancer.

During this week, you'll make solid sleep a priority, with the foods you choose, the activities you undertake and the changes you make to your sleep routine. I promise within just a few days, you'll see an incredible difference in how you sleep at night—and how you feel all day. And even after the program ends, you'll have set the stage for the sleep that will give you power, energy and vitality for the days, months and years to come.

PART THREE

THE THREE-WEEK PLAN

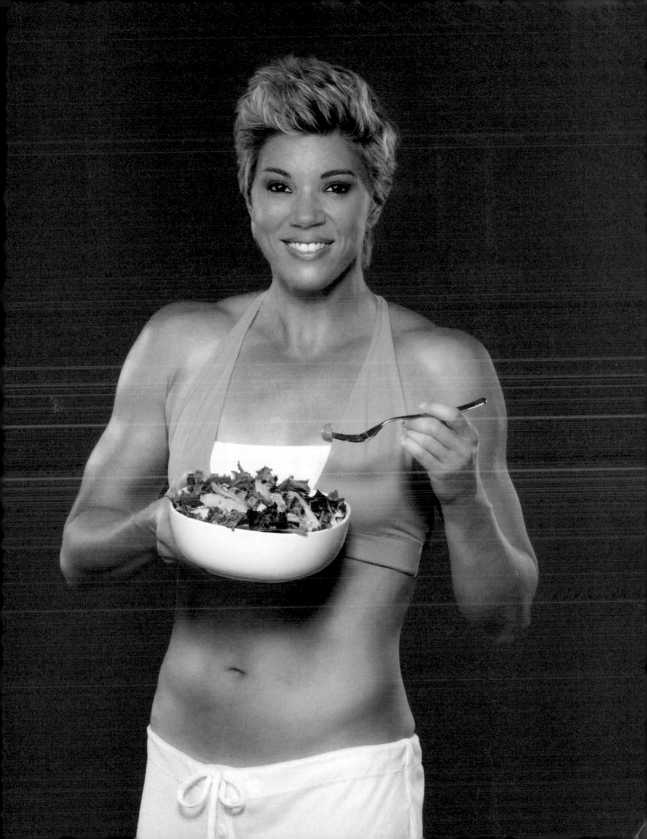

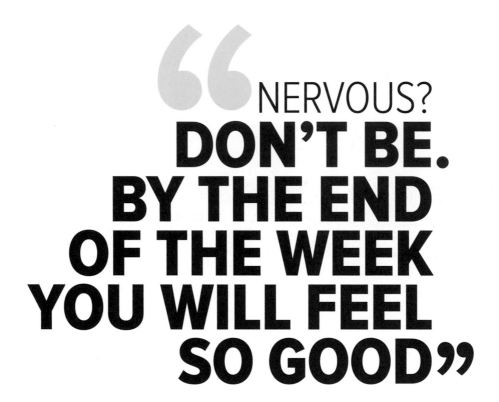

"NERVOUS?
DON'T BE.
BY THE END
OF THE WEEK
YOU WILL FEEL
SO GOOD"

CHAPTER SEVEN

PHASE ONE: DETOX & PRIME

During this week, you're going to rebuild your body's cells and glands. Prepare to go on the king of all cleanses because it is the most thorough and *only* way to do a cleanse right. Forget what you've heard about cleanses where you drink nothing but maple syrup and cayenne pepper; a cleanse should consist of several nutrient-dense whole foods, not just juices. Drinking a liquid-only diet causes such starvation that you can permanently slow down your metabolism and throw your system completely out of balance. Then when you introduce solid foods, you can actually gain weight. A proper cleanse should give you much more energy, not make you feel like you have the flu!

As part of the cleanse, I'm also going to ask you to remove all negative crutches that you may be abusing just in this first week. Let's give your body a chance to feel pure and run efficiently. So this means removing the following crutches from your diet:

* Coffee
* "Energy" drinks
* Refined sugar
* Alcohol
* Medications not used for treatment of a serious condition
* Marijuana

Nervous? Don't be. By the end of the week you will feel so good that it will out-weigh the temporary fix you may have got from the list above. The foods I have chosen for you are so energizing that you should feel better almost instantly.

During the detox, you'll drink three liters of cold water every day. Cold water gives you an energy boost as well as detoxifies your organs and cells. If you are trying to lose weight, water is your best ally—drinking three liters a day will speed up your metabolism significantly. I'm also including my secret weapon against sickness and aging—an amazing detox tea made of ginger. You will make a batch that lasts you three days and you should drink it every night for weight loss, beautiful skin and strong immunity! The act of drinking tea satisfies an oral fixation and it's important that you have a healthy substitute for the bad drinks I'm asking you to forgo.

PHASE 1: BETTER SLEEP

In the previous chapter you learned all about how to get better-quality sleep. Start making those lifestyle changes—going to bed and getting up at the same time, keeping your room dark and cool, "unplugging" well before bedtime—now, during Phase 1. As you go forward, the 21-Day Detox diet and the workout plan will support your lifestyle changes, leading to the best sleep of your life!

BREAKING BAD HABITS

Many of you will go through emotional withdrawals without your negative coping crutches. Remember, don't be hard on yourself. The brain is designed to be addicted to chemicals that stimulate its pleasure centers. Of course we gravitate toward foods and substances that spike serotonin (the feel-good chemical of the brain). I fully understand because I cut out all alcohol for a year myself. I realized that I got quite dependent on my nightly glass of wine at the end of the day and before I knew it, one had turned to three.

Alcohol is highly addictive, and if you make it part of your regular routine, your brain will want more as time goes on. I know all about brain chemistry and I knew that I had to stop the bad habit. I knew that my excessive drinking was unhealthy and I quit, thus allowing my brain to reset itself as well as giving a lot of thought to why I was looking to check out at night. We turn to serotonin releasers, such as fatty and sugary foods, alcohol, cigarettes and marijuana, in order to deal with stress, boredom and frustration.

I have to share with you that initially it was difficult not being able to unwind with a drink. But the personal growth and vitality that came from abstaining changed the whole trajectory of my life. I found that I had a clarity of mind and strength of body to start a new chapter in life. I started painting again and selling my work, I fulfilled a lifelong dream of starting a band and I created new television projects that I was truly passionate about!

All my personal relationships greatly improved because I was fully present and engaged with everyone around me—in general, my personality became much more vibrant. Without crutches to artificially keep me from feeling, my mind was forced to work all by itself in dealing with pain and stress. A longtime resentment I had with my mother completely healed and now she is my best friend and we talk for an hour or more every day.

You find out what you're made of when you are forced to deal with life in full reality, only using positive things to stimulate yourself. An inner strength that you never knew you had will emerge and it will build tremendous self-esteem. When you make good choices for yourself, good things come to you! If you decide to continue past the seven-day detox program without addictive substances, I highly suggest that you start a journal and write down your feelings each day as you journey to the greatest version of you.

PHASE 1: DETOX

The first seven days of this program, Phase 1, will be an almost exclusively vegan cleanse; you will not consume animal proteins (other than the minimal amounts of dairy products contained in whole-grain bread and pasta). This will be your base diet for the 21-day program. Each seven days, you will simply build on these detox meals. Each meal will consist of whole fruits or vegetables and a whole grain and healthy fat. You will get your protein mainly through nuts, seeds, legumes and grains. I've structured the first seven days of the plan to provide 1,300–1,550 calories a day. Your daily breakfast contains about 300–350 calories; each snack 150–200 calories; lunch 300–350 calories; and dinner 400–450 calories.

You will have plenty of energy to perform the prime workouts for this week, which are relatively light and meant to teach you technique. If you feel a craving in the first couple of days, just remind yourself that you are truly nourishing your body. I promise by midweek you'll feel more energetic, upbeat and healthy.

Weight Loss

If you're looking to lose weight with this program, trust me—you will! All foods included in this plan, even at the higher calorie range, are extreme fat-burners that have been carefully chosen to help you lean out. Science now tells us that it's not only the number of calories you consume—it's the *quality* of those calories that makes a difference in your health. And research proves that consuming nutrient-dense but lower-calorie foods, like the fruits and vegetables this diet is based on, assists not only with weight loss but keeping those pounds off for good. Highly nutrient-dense foods react entirely differently in your body and actually speed metabolism and cause a fat-burning environment, even when you're consuming more calories.

On this plan, you'll eat the following foods that detoxify and support your cells, glands, immune function and skin. The starred ingredients will be incorporated in all three weeks of the program, but if you decide to substitute foods, feel free to consume anything on the list on the next page:

Almonds*	Fava beans	Peanuts*
Apples*	Flaxseeds/flaxseed oil*	Pears*
Apricots	Garlic*	Peas*
Asparagus*	Grapefruits*	Pecans*
Avocados*	Green tea*	Pine nuts*
Bananas*	Guava	Pinto beans*
Beans	Hazelnuts	Pistachios*
Bell peppers*	Honey*	Potatoes*
Blackberries*	Kale*	Prunes
Brazil nuts	Kiwifruit	Pumpkin seeds*
Broccoli*	Lentils*	Raspberries*
Brown rice*	Lima beans	Red cabbage
Brussels sprouts	Melons*	Sesame seeds*
Butternut squash*	Mung beans	Spinach*
Cantaloupe*	Mushrooms*	Strawberries*
Carrots*	Navy beans*	Sun-dried tomatoes*
Cauliflower*	Nectarines*	Sunflower seeds*
Cherries*	Olive oil*	Sweet potatoes*
Chickpeas*	Oats (steel-cut, whole)*	Swiss chard
Chili peppers, red and green	Onions*	Tomatoes*
Coconut oil*	Oranges*	Turnip greens
Collard greens	Quinoa*	Walnuts*
Corn*	Papayas*	Watermelon*

On this plan, you'll eat five times a day: breakfast, a midmorning snack, lunch, an afternoon snack and dinner. I've made it easy for you by choosing meals and snacks that contain the highest amount of nutrients that you need to cleanse, detox and rebuild your body's polluted, overworked cells. In the pages that follow, you'll find:

- 21 breakfast power smoothie options
- 21 snack options
- 21 lunch options
- 21 dinner options

Each day, you'll choose one meal and two snacks from each of the four categories; the choice is yours. All I ask is that each day you choose something different for each of the five meals to ensure a wide balance of the necessary nutrients for cellular detox and health. Ready? Let's start with breakfast!

The Calorie Boost

If you are relatively fit and already exercise a fair amount, then this phase of the program may not provide enough calories for you. If so, I recommend a "Calorie Boost." Each day, simply add 10 nuts and an additional portable fruit to your meals and snacks. Consume your Calorie Boost when you feel the hungriest.

The Well-Stocked Pantry (and Fridge)

If you jump ahead and scan through the recipes, you'll see that they feature a wide range of ingredients to ensure that your cells get the detoxifying nutrients you need. However, to follow the program, it helps to always have some of the "basics" on hand. Here are some of the foods that are used frequently in recipes, and that I suggest you keep in your pantry, refrigerator and freezer.

Pantry

- ☐ Almond butter
- ☐ Almonds
- ☐ Bananas
- ☐ Black beans (canned)
- ☐ Black olives (canned)
- ☐ Chickpeas (canned)
- ☐ Chili powder
- ☐ Corn (canned)
- ☐ Cumin
- ☐ Extra-virgin olive oil
- ☐ Flaxseed oil
- ☐ Instant brown rice
- ☐ Instant oats (look for a large package, not the single-serve ones)
- ☐ Pepper
- ☐ Pineapple (canned, no sugar added)
- ☐ Pine nuts
- ☐ Quinoa
- ☐ Rice cakes
- ☐ Sea salt
- ☐ Sesame seeds
- ☐ Sun-dried tomatoes in oil
- ☐ Walnuts
- ☐ Whole-grain bread
- ☐ Whole-grain pasta
- ☐ Whole-grain tortillas (6-inch size)

Refrigerator

- ☐ Avocados
- ☐ Bean sprouts
- ☐ Blueberries
- ☐ Broccoli
- ☐ Carrots
- ☐ Celery
- ☐ Garlic
- ☐ Ginger (for tea)
- ☐ Grapefruits
- ☐ Grapes
- ☐ Kale
- ☐ Mangos
- ☐ Mixed greens
- ☐ Onions
- ☐ Oranges
- ☐ Pears
- ☐ Peppers (sweet red)
- ☐ Romaine lettuce
- ☐ Spinach
- ☐ Strawberries
- ☐ Sweet potatoes
- ☐ Tomatoes
- ☐ Unsweetened almond milk

Freezer

- ☐ Frozen blueberries (no sugar added)
- ☐ Frozen mixed berries (no sugar added)
- ☐ Frozen strawberries (no sugar added)

WHAT YOU'LL NEED TO GET STARTED

- Blender

- Measuring cup

- Steamer

The easiest and quickest way to consume the right amount of whole fruits and veggies is by blending them into delicious power smoothies. During the detox, breakfasts will always be blended and contain a sizable portion of your nutrients. These are not just smoothies; these are complete meals that should sustain you for hours. I have given you 21 power smoothies to choose from. It's actually a lot of fun to try all of them to see which ones you love. The key is to drink a variety of shakes so that you get a wide range of healing nutrients.

In addition to the blender, buy a "drop-in" metal steamer that sits in a cooking pot. These inexpensive steamers can be found at most kitchen or housewares stores and will help you get the most nutrients out of your veggies. Grab a measuring cup to get you started, but by the end of the week you should be able to "eye" the portions without the cup.

Ginger Detox Tea

I absolutely love this immunity-building detox tea. Make a big pot every three days, keep it in your fridge and drink it at night instead of snacking. Slice 4 large (three to four inches across) pieces of fresh ginger (no peeling necessary) and add to 6 cups of water and 4 tablespoons of lemon juice. Boil for 30 minutes. To drink, strain into a cup, reheat and add a bag of decaffeinated green tea.

BREAKFAST OPTIONS

I love power smoothies for breakfast because they're fast, convenient and delicious—while loaded with the nutrients you need for the optimal detox. Have fun trying different ones and deciding which you like the best. Each smoothie recipe here contains some whole oats and healthy fat in the form of flaxseed oil for satiety and energy, and has between 300 and 360 calories. Look for "instant oats" on the package; these come in a large container that you can measure from, not the prepackaged, presweetened single-serve oatmeal packets.

Each smoothie also contains a mix of fruits and/or vegetables. You can use either fresh or frozen fruit in your smoothie, although I suggest frozen because it is slightly higher in nutrients as it's frozen immediately after picking. Just make sure you're buying fruit that doesn't have any sugar added to it. Whenever possible, choose organic fruits and vegetables to avoid pesticides and other toxins. If you use frozen fruit, you don't need to add the extra ice called for in the recipe.

While an ordinary blender will work fine, you may want to consider investing in a top-line model such as a Vitamix. It has a single-serve smoothie cup and takes only a few seconds to use and rinse out. You should consume your smoothie as soon as you get up to jump-start your metabolism.

The Science Behind My Power Smoothies

My smoothies are not your average smoothie. They are packed with the essential nutrients that balance blood sugar, elevate energy and fight disease. Notice that flaxseed oil and oats are included in each one to fill you up and give you a dose of healthy fat and whole grains. Healthy fats, like flaxseed oil, are essential for cellular function and overall health, and help keep you feeling satisfied between meals. And the whole grains contained in oatmeal provide fiber, another proven weight-loss tool, which also helps "power" you through your morning. Each recipe makes one serving.

Berry Smoothie

1 cup mixed berries

1 cup fresh spinach

1 tablespoon almond butter

¼ cup instant oats

1 tablespoon flaxseed oil

½ cup water

Combine all ingredients and blend well.

341 CALORIES

Pineapple Smoothie

1 cup pineapple

½ banana

½ cup unsweetened almond milk

¼ cup instant oats

1 tablespoon flaxseed oil

½ cup ice

¼ cup water

Combine all ingredients and blend well.

360 CALORIES

Citrus Smoothie

1 medium grapefruit, peeled and sectioned

1 banana

½ cup unsweetened almond milk

¼ cup instant oats

1 tablespoon flaxseed oil

½ cup ice

Combine all ingredients and blend well.

347 CALORIES

Beet Smoothie

1 fresh, cooked (or canned) beet, sliced thin

1 cup cherries, pitted

½ cup unsweetened almond milk

¼ cup instant oats

1 tablespoon flaxseed oil

½ cup ice

Combine all ingredients and blend well.

300 CALORIES

Orange Smoothie

1 medium orange, peeled and sectioned

½ small banana

½ cup unsweetened almond milk

¼ cup instant oats

1 tablespoon flaxseed oil

1 cup ice

Combine all ingredients and blend well.

322 CALORIES

Blueberry-Banana Smoothie

1 cup blueberries

½ banana

½ cup unsweetened almond milk

¼ cup instant oats

1 tablespoon flaxseed oil

½ cup ice

Combine all ingredients and blend well.

327 CALORIES

Strawberries and Chocolate Smoothie

1 cup strawberries

1 tablespoon unsweetened cocoa powder

1 tablespoon honey

½ cup unsweetened almond milk

¼ cup instant oats

1 tablespoon flaxseed oil

½ cup ice

Combine all ingredients and blend well.

314 CALORIES

Melon Smoothie

1 cup cantaloupe, cubed

1 cup strawberries

½ cup unsweetened almond milk

¼ cup instant oats

1 tablespoon flaxseed oil

½ cup ice

Combine all ingredients and blend well.

346 CALORIES

Apple Smoothie

1 medium apple, cored and coarsely chopped

1 cup fresh spinach

½ cup unsweetened almond milk

¼ cup instant oats

1 tablespoon flaxseed oil

½ cup ice

Combine all ingredients and blend well.

330 CALORIES

Grape-Lime Smoothie

2 cups green grapes

1 tablespoon lime juice

1 cup fresh spinach

½ cup unsweetened almond milk

¼ cup instant oats

1 tablespoon flaxseed oil

Combine all ingredients and blend well.

320 CALORIES

Avocado-Pear Smoothie

½ avocado, pitted, peeled and cut into chunks

½ medium pear, cut into chunks

¼ cup instant oats

1 tablespoon flaxseed oil

1 cup ice

¼ cup water

Combine all ingredients and blend well.

338 CALORIES

Pineapple– Mixed Berry Smoothie

1 cup pineapple, cubed

1 cup mixed berries

½ cup unsweetened almond milk

¼ cup instant oats

1 tablespoon flaxseed oil

1 cup ice

Combine all ingredients and blend well.

340 CALORIES

Super-Antioxidant Smoothie

1 cup cranberries

1 cup mixed berries

1 cup fresh spinach

½ cup unsweetened almond milk

¼ cup instant oats

1 tablespoon flaxseed oil

½ cup water

Combine all ingredients and blend well.

311 CALORIES

Carrot-Orange Smoothie

1 carrot, chopped

1 medium orange, peeled and sectioned

1 cup fresh spinach

½ cup unsweetened almond milk

¼ cup instant oats

1 tablespoon flaxseed oil

½ cup ice

Combine all ingredients and blend well.

300 CALORIES

Mango-Strawberry Smoothie

1 ½ cups mango chunks

1 cup strawberries

½ cup unsweetened almond milk

¼ cup instant oats

1 tablespoon flaxseed oil

½ cup water

Combine all ingredients and blend well.

338 CALORIES

Banana-Avocado Smoothie

½ medium banana

½ avocado, pitted, peeled and cut into chunks

1 cup fresh spinach

2 tablespoons lime juice

¼ cup instant oats

1 tablespoon flaxseed oil

Dash of water

Combine all ingredients and blend well.

350 CALORIES

Cran-Blueberry Smoothie

1 cup cranberries

1 cup blueberries

½ cup almond milk

¼ cup instant oats

1 tablespoon flaxseed oil

½ cup water

Combine all ingredients and blend well.

321 CALORIES

Apple Pie Smoothie

1 ½ medium apples, chopped into chunks

½ teaspoon cinnamon

⅓ teaspoon nutmeg

½ teaspoon 100 percent pure vanilla extract

½ cup unsweetened almond milk

½ cup instant oats

1 tablespoon flaxseed oil

¼ cup ice

Combine all ingredients and blend well.

332 CALORIES

Cherry- Grapefruit Smoothie

1 cup cherries, pitted

1 medium grapefruit, peeled and sectioned

¼ cup instant oats

½ cup unsweetened almond milk

1 tablespoon flaxseed oil

1 cup water

Combine all ingredients and blend well.

319 CALORIES

Aloha Smoothie

1 cup mango, peeled and chopped

½ cup pineapple

½ cup unsweetened almond milk

¼ cup instant oats

1 tablespoon flaxseed oil

1 cup ice

Combine all ingredients and blend well.

333 CALORIES

Super Spinach Smoothie

2 cups fresh spinach

4 strawberries

1 banana

½ cup instant oats

1 tablespoon flaxseed oil

½ cup ice

Combine all ingredients and blend well.

----

304 CALORIES

TIP

Toasted nuts give a flavor boost and crunch.

Roasting nuts in the oven will deepen and bring out their flavor. To roast them, preheat your oven to 350°F. Toss the nuts lightly with coconut or olive oil, spread them on a baking pan and bake for five minutes. Move the nuts from the outside of the pan to the inside, and vice versa, for even roasting, and put them back in for another three minutes or so. Check the nuts for doneness; they're roasted when they're a few shades darker than they were. Be careful to watch them carefully and not to overcook them. They can burn quickly.

Try roasting:

- sesame seeds
- walnuts
- almonds
- pumpkin seeds
- pine nuts (my fave!)

Make a bunch and keep them in an airtight container until you're ready to use them.

SNACK OPTIONS

Snacks are meant to keep your blood sugar balanced until you have your next complete meal. I find that a snack between breakfast and lunch and another in midafternoon helps keep my energy levels high. Snacks also prevent you from going too long between meals; you do not want to skip your snack because when your blood sugar plummets, the next thing you put in your mouth is almost twice as effectively stored as fat.

Here are some quick and easy snack options that you can put in a plastic storage container and take to work or eat at home. The majority of your snacks include a fruit with nuts or seeds. The key to a good snack is portability. Place your toasted nuts and seeds in small plastic bags or containers and simply take them with you.

Just as you did with breakfast, choose a different snack each day to ensure that you're getting a variety of nutrients. Each includes some healthy fat, protein and carbs to give you sustained energy.

Nutty Melon

2 cups watermelon and cantaloupe, sliced into chunks

4 teaspoons pine nuts, toasted

Sprinkle toasted pine nuts on top and eat.

MAKES 1 SERVING 166 CALORIES

Carrots/Celery and Hummus

10 baby carrots or 3 stalks celery

¼ cup store-bought hummus (or see recipe on page 158)

Dip and eat. For variety, try sliced cucumbers, fresh broccoli or cauliflower instead.

MAKES 1 SERVING 185 CALORIES

Baba Ghanoush and Cucumber

1 large cucumber, sliced

1 cup prepared baba ghanoush (or make your own—see recipe below)

Dip and eat.

MAKES 1 SERVING **170 CALORIES**

Baba Ghanoush

1 medium-sized eggplant

1 tablespoon extra-virgin olive oil

2 tablespoons lemon juice

1 tablespoon tahini

1 tablespoon garlic, minced

½ teaspoon paprika

¼ teaspoon sea salt

3 tablespoons parsley, chopped

Preheat oven to 450°F.

Prick the eggplant all over with a fork and place on an oiled baking sheet. Roast for 20 minutes or until soft.

In a blender or food processor, combine eggplant and olive oil, lemon juice, tahini, garlic, paprika and salt until smooth. You may need to add more or less oil and lemon juice in order to get the proper consistency.

Stir in parsley.

MAKES ABOUT 2 SERVINGS
150 CALORIES EACH

Almond Butter and Celery

2 tablespoons almond butter

2 large celery stalks

Spread almond butter over celery stalks and eat.

MAKES 1 SERVING **190 CALORIES**

Tomato with Pine Nuts

2 tablespoons pine nuts, toasted

1 tablespoon balsamic vinegar

1 large tomato, sliced

Sprinkle pine nuts and balsamic vinegar on tomato slices before eating.

MAKES 1 SERVING **182 CALORIES**

Peanut Butter and Banana Rice Cake

1 tablespoon peanut butter

1 plain rice cake

½ small banana, sliced

Spread peanut butter onto rice cake and top with banana slices.

MAKES 1 SERVING **175 CALORIES**

Baked Chips with Pico de Gallo

15 store-bought baked tortilla chips (or make your own—see recipe below)

½ cup premade or homemade Pico de Gallo (see recipe on page 166)

2 slices avocado, cut in pieces

Dip chips in Pico de Gallo, and top with a small piece of avocado.

MAKES 1 SERVING 188 CALORIES

Skinny Tortilla Chips

Small corn tortillas (6-inch size)

Canola oil cooking spray

Sea salt

Preheat oven to 350°F.

Lightly spray each side of the tortillas before stacking them on top of each other and slicing into 8 pieces (like a pizza). Sprinkle tortilla pieces with salt and place them on baking sheets; bake for 10–12 minutes until they are lightly browned and crisp. They will curl slightly as they bake.

----

45 CALORIES EACH

Spicy Toasted Chickpeas

1 fifteen-ounce can chickpeas, drained and rinsed

2 tablespoons extra-virgin olive oil

1 teaspoon cumin

1 teaspoon chili powder

1 teaspoon garlic salt

Preheat oven to 450°F.

Dry chickpeas with a towel or a paper towel. Toss chickpeas with olive oil and spread on a baking sheet. Mix cumin, chili powder and garlic salt, and sprinkle over chickpeas; bake for 30–40 minutes, stirring several times to avoid burning. Remove when brown and crunchy.

**MAKES 4 SERVINGS
181 CALORIES EACH**

Almond-Kale Chips

1 large bunch kale, washed and torn into chip-sized pieces

1 tablespoon extra-virgin olive oil

½ teaspoon garlic powder

Sea salt

1 teaspoon crushed toasted almonds

Preheat oven to 375°F.

Pat kale leaves dry and spread them out on a baking sheet. Drizzle with olive oil and sprinkle with garlic powder, salt and almonds; bake for about 10–15 minutes or until chips are crisp.

MAKES 2 SERVINGS
146 CALORIES EACH

Coconut Pineapple

5 macadamia nuts, chopped

¾ cup pineapple chunks

1 tablespoon unsweetened shredded coconut

Combine nuts and pineapple in a bowl and sprinkle with coconut.

MAKES 1 SERVING 177 CALORIES

Honey Pear

1 pear, cut into chunks

1 teaspoon honey

1 tablespoon pumpkin seeds, toasted

Mix pear with honey in a bowl. Top with toasted seeds.

MAKES 1 SERVING 182 CALORIES

Bell Peppers with Sweet Potato Hummus

2 medium sweet potatoes (about 2 cups)

⅛ cup tahini

⅛ cup fresh lime juice

1 teaspoon garlic, minced

1 teaspoon cumin

1 teaspoon sea salt

Cayenne pepper, to taste

1 bell pepper, sliced

Peel and chop sweet potatoes into small (about 1-inch) chunks. Using a steamer, steam potatoes until soft (about 15–20 minutes).

Place potato chunks, tahini, lime juice, garlic, cumin, salt and a few shakes of cayenne pepper into a blender or food processor and blend until creamy.

Serve with bell pepper.

MAKES 4 SERVINGS
153 CALORIES EACH

Frozen Grapes with Pumpkin Seeds

½ cup frozen grapes

2 tablespoons roasted pumpkin seeds

Freeze grapes overnight before mixing with roasted pumpkin seeds.

MAKES 1 SERVING 162 CALORIES

Peach Bread

2 teaspoons all-natural almond butter

1 slice whole-grain bread, toasted

½ peach, sliced

Spread almond butter on toasted bread and top with peach slices.

MAKES 1 SERVING 163 CALORIES

Spicy Avocado

1 teaspoon lime juice

Sriracha or other chili sauce

½ avocado, peeled with the pit removed

1 teaspoon almonds, slivered

Drizzle lime juice and sriracha sauce over avocado and sprinkle with almonds.

MAKES 1 SERVING 157 CALORIES

Cinnamon-Apple Slices

1 teaspoon honey

1 apple, cored and thinly sliced

1 tablespoon almonds, toasted and chopped

Sprinkle of cinnamon

Drizzle honey over apple slices and top with almonds and a sprinkle of cinnamon.

MAKES 1 SERVING 172 CALORIES

Quick Wrap

2 tablespoons prepared hummus or sweet potato hummus (see recipe on page 158)

1 whole-grain tortilla (6-inch size)

1 drizzle extra-virgin olive oil

Spread hummus on tortilla and drizzle olive oil on top.

MAKES 1 SERVING 150 CALORIES

Strawberry– Almond Butter Rice Cake

1 tablespoon all-natural almond butter

1 plain rice cake

4 strawberries, sliced

Cinnamon

Spread almond butter on rice cake and top with sliced strawberries. Sprinkle with cinnamon.

MAKES 1 SERVING 151 CALORIES

Almond Butter and Coconut Apple

1 apple

2 teaspoons all-natural almond butter

1 teaspoon unsweetened shredded coconut

Cut apple in half and core. Spread almond butter over halves and sprinkle with coconut.

MAKES 1 SERVING 169 CALORIES

Guacamole and Chips

½ avocado, cored and peeled

1 tablespoon finely chopped onion

½ teaspoon garlic, minced

¼ cup chopped tomato

1 teaspoon lime juice

Sea salt

Pepper

10 baked tortilla chips
(see recipe on page 157)

Use a potato masher to mash the avocado in a medium-sized bowl. Add onion, garlic, tomato and lime juice; add salt and pepper to taste. Serve with tortilla chips.

MAKES 1 SERVING 182 CALORIES

Artichoke Dip

1 nine-ounce box frozen artichoke hearts, thawed and chopped

1/2 cup sun-dried tomatoes in oil, chopped

1/4 cup pine nuts, toasted

1 tablespoon garlic, minced

2 teaspoons lemon juice

Sea salt

Pepper

4 cups broccoli florets or sliced bell peppers

In a food processor or blender, combine artichokes, tomatoes, pine nuts, garlic and lemon juice. Add salt and pepper to taste. Serve with broccoli florets or sliced bell peppers or carrots.

MAKES 4 SERVINGS, EACH WITH 1 CUP OF FRESH VEGETABLES 162 CALORIES EACH

LUNCH OPTIONS

The lunch options I've chosen are simple but delicious. All recipes here are easy and portable. Your lunches will consist of:

- Salads

- Sandwiches

- Wraps

Each lunch has multiple nutrients to deliver a huge nutritional impact, but none of these meals should take more than 10 minutes for prep and cooking. Just as with the power smoothies, choose one from this list for each day so that you try seven different meals. Many of these recipes include whole grains, such as brown rice, couscous or quinoa, which are loaded with nutrients and fiber. These meals will give you sustained energy for even the most demanding of afternoons!

Cook Once, Eat Often

Here's a tip: choose a weekend afternoon or evening and cook a batch or two of your favorite grain, whether quinoa or brown rice, and store the cooked grains in a storage container in the fridge for quick meal prep.

SUPER SALAD DRESSINGS

Forget the packaged salad dressings that you find in the store. I've created salad dressings for the detox diet that are loaded with cell-boosting nutrients, minus anything artificial. For your convenience, I've listed them all here; if you find a favorite, mix up a batch of it and keep it in your refrigerator as your go-to dressing.

Fresh Orange Dressing

1/4 cup fresh orange juice

1 tablespoon red wine vinegar

2 tablespoons extra-virgin olive oil

1 tablespoon basil, chopped

Combine all ingredients in a glass jar or blender and shake or process until smooth. Store in a glass jar in the refrigerator.

MAKES 7 ONE-TABLESPOON SERVINGS
100 CALORIES EACH

Garlic Salad Dressing

¼ cup extra-virgin olive oil

1 tablespoon garlic, minced

1 tablespoon lemon juice

1 teaspoon fresh thyme or basil, chopped

Dash of sea salt

Dash of pepper

Combine all ingredients in a glass jar or blender and shake or process until smooth. Store in a glass jar in the refrigerator.

MAKES 7 ONE-TABLESPOON SERVINGS
115 CALORIES EACH

Peanut Dressing

2 tablespoons sesame oil

1 tablespoon lemon juice, fresh squeezed

1 tablespoon honey or agave nectar

1 tablespoon soy sauce

1 teaspoon ginger, grated

1 tablespoon peanut butter

Combine all ingredients in a glass jar or blender and shake or process until smooth. Store in a glass jar in the refrigerator.

MAKES 6 ONE-TABLESPOON SERVINGS
70 CALORIES EACH

Greek Salad Dressing

¼ cup extra-virgin olive oil

1 tablespoon basil

1 teaspoon garlic, minced

¼ teaspoon onion powder

1 teaspoon Dijon mustard

1 teaspoon fresh black pepper

Dash of sea salt

2 tablespoons red wine vinegar

Combine all ingredients in a glass jar or blender and shake or process until smooth. Store in a glass jar in the refrigerator.

MAKES 10 ONE-TABLESPOON SERVINGS
110 CALORIES EACH

Mustard Vinaigrette Dressing

¼ cup extra-virgin olive oil

¼ cup balsamic vinegar

½ teaspoon garlic, minced

½ teaspoon ground mustard

¼ teaspoon pepper

Sea salt

Combine all ingredients in a glass jar or blender and shake or process until smooth. Store in a glass jar in the refrigerator.

MAKES 10 ONE-TABLESPOON SERVINGS
70 CALORIES EACH

Herb Vinaigrette Dressing

2 ½ tablespoons extra-virgin olive oil

1 tablespoon Herbs de Provence

1 teaspoon garlic, minced

1 ½ tablespoons balsamic vinegar

Dash each, sea salt and pepper

Combine all ingredients in a glass jar or blender and shake or process until smooth. Store in a glass jar in the refrigerator.

MAKES 5 ONE-TABLESPOON SERVINGS
ABOUT 100 CALORIES EACH

Cilantro-Lime Dressing

2 tablespoons extra-virgin olive oil

1 teaspoon fresh lime juice

½ teaspoon cilantro

Dash sriracha sauce

Combine all ingredients in a glass jar or blender and shake or process until smooth. Store in a glass jar in the refrigerator.

MAKES 2 ONE-TABLESPOON SERVINGS
85 CALORIES EACH

Asian Salad Dressing

2 tablespoons extra-virgin olive oil

1 tablespoon soy sauce (low-sodium, if possible)

1 tablespoon rice wine vinegar (or white vinegar)

¼ teaspoon red pepper flakes

1 teaspoon sesame seeds, toasted

Combine all ingredients in a glass jar or blender and shake or process until smooth. Store in a glass jar in the refrigerator.

MAKES 4 ONE-TABLESPOON SERVINGS
75 CALORIES EACH

Lemon-Paprika Dressing

2 tablespoons extra-virgin olive oil

1 teaspoon lemon juice

1 teaspoon garlic, minced

½ teaspoon paprika

2 tablespoons extra-virgin olive oil

Combine all ingredients in a glass jar or blender and shake or process until smooth. Store in a glass jar in the refrigerator.

MAKES 3 ONE-TABLESPOON SERVINGS
85 CALORIES EACH

Sun-Dried Tomato Hummus Sandwich

¼ cup store-bought Sun-Dried Tomato Hummus
(or see recipe, this page)

2 slices whole-grain bread

1 slice onion

3 leaves romaine lettuce

½ tomato, sliced

½ cup alfalfa or bean sprouts

Sea salt

Pepper

Spread hummus over 1 slice of bread. Top with onion, lettuce, tomato and sprouts, and sprinkle with salt and pepper to taste before topping with the other slice of bread.

MAKES 1 SERVING 340 CALORIES

Sun-Dried Tomato Hummus

2 tablespoons extra-virgin olive oil

1 teaspoon garlic, minced

1 fifteen-ounce can garbanzo beans

4 tablespoons lemon juice

2 tablespoons sun-dried tomatoes, packed in oil

1 teaspoon sea salt

1 tablespoon tahini

Place all ingredients in a blender or food processor and blend until creamy.

**MAKES ABOUT 4 SERVINGS
160 CALORIES EACH**

Garlic Crouton Recipe

Add some crunch and extra satisfaction to your salads with my simple garlic crouton recipe:

½ loaf whole grain bread

garlic powder

2 tablespoons extra-virgin olive oil

Preheat oven to 400°F. Cut bread into ¼-inch cubes. Brush bread cubes with oil and sprinkle garlic powder on top. Spread in a rimmed baking pan and bake until brown and crisp, turning frequently.

Store in a container or a resealable plastic bag to maintain crispiness.

Orange-Strawberry Salad

3 cups mixed greens

1 cup sliced strawberries

½ orange, cut into small segments

1 green onion, sliced

2 tablespoons sliced almonds

10 Garlic Croutons (see recipe on page 164)

1 tablespoon Fresh Orange Dressing (see recipe on page 162)

In a medium bowl, add the first 5 ingredients. Toss well with dressing and top with croutons.

MAKES 1 SERVING 330 CALORIES

Chopped Italian Salad

3 cups or 1 bunch lettuce, chopped

1 cup cherry tomatoes, halved

1 green bell pepper, seeded and diced into small pieces

½ red onion, diced small

¼ cup Kalamata olives, pitted and chopped

1 tablespoon fresh basil, chopped fine

2 peppercinis, diced

2 tablespoons pine nuts, toasted

Sea salt and pepper to taste

1 tablespoon Garlic Salad Dressing (see recipe on page 162)

10 Garlic Croutons

In a medium bowl, add the first 8 ingredients and season with salt and pepper. Toss well with dressing and top with croutons.

MAKES 1 SERVING 330 CALORIES

Asian Peanut Salad

3 cups mixed greens

2 carrots, grated

1 red pepper, finely diced

2 celery stalks, finely diced

¼ medium red onion, finely diced

¼ cup cilantro, chopped

⅛ cup roasted peanuts, chopped

10 Garlic Croutons (see recipe on page 164)

1 tablespoon Peanut Dressing (see recipe on page 162)

In a medium bowl, add the first 7 ingredients. Toss well with dressing and top with croutons.

MAKES 1 SERVING 322 CALORIES

Greek Wrap

1 cup romaine lettuce, finely chopped

2 slices red onion

½ cup chopped cucumber

½ cup cherry tomatoes, chopped

¼ cup Kalamata olives, diced small

Greek Salad Dressing (see recipe on page 162)

Oregano, sea salt and pepper to taste

2 tablespoons prepared hummus

1 whole-grain tortilla (6-inch size)

In a small bowl, toss lettuce, red onion, cucumber, cherry tomatoes and olives with 1 tablespoon of dressing. Add oregano, salt and pepper to taste. Spread hummus over tortilla and top with veggie mixture. Drizzle more dressing on top; roll up tortilla before eating.

MAKES 1 SERVING 320 CALORIES

Guacamole Wrap

½ avocado, thinly sliced

½ tomato, chopped

½ red onion, chopped

1 teaspoon lemon juice

1 teaspoon extra-virgin olive oil

Coriander

Sea salt

Pepper

1 whole-grain tortilla (6-inch size)

1 teaspoon pine nuts

1 tablespoon Pico de Gallo (see recipe below)

Place the avocado, tomato and red onion on a cutting board and drizzle with lemon juice and olive oil. Top with coriander. Add salt and pepper to taste. Toss well. Place mixture on tortilla and top with pine nuts and Pico de Gallo; roll up the tortilla before eating.

MAKES 1 SERVING 320 CALORIES

Pico de Gallo

2 medium tomatoes, diced

1 small onion, chopped fine

½ jalapeño pepper, seeded and chopped

1 green onion, chopped fine

½ teaspoon garlic powder

⅛ teaspoon sea salt

Pepper to taste

Blend all ingredients. Chill before serving.

MAKES ABOUT 2 SERVINGS 30 CALORIES EACH

Pear and Bell Pepper Salad

½ sweet red pepper, cored and seeded

½ sweet yellow pepper, cored and seeded

¼ cup green onion

1 medium pear, peeled

Sea salt

Pepper

1 teaspoon rice vinegar

1 teaspoon sesame oil

2 cups mixed greens

1 tablespoon Herb Vinaigrette Dressing or Fresh Orange Dressing (see recipes on pages 163 and 162)

¼ cup fresh parsley or fresh basil leaves, chopped

3 tablespoons pine nuts, toasted

10 Garlic Croutons (see recipe on page 164)

Slice peppers, onions and pear into thin strips and place in a shallow bowl. Sprinkle with salt and pepper. Spoon rice vinegar and sesame oil over mixture and place mixed greens on top.

Top salad with dressing, chopped parsley or basil, pine nuts and croutons.

MAKES 1 SERVING 313 CALORIES

Strawberry and Kale Salad

3 cups baby kale, chopped

10 strawberries, sliced

1 medium tomato, chopped

1 tablespoon Mustard Vinaigrette Dressing (see recipe on page 163)

2 tablespoons walnuts, toasted and chopped

Place kale, strawberries and tomato in a medium bowl and toss with dressing. Top with toasted walnuts.

MAKES 1 SERVING 341 CALORIES

Artichoke Salad

1 cup artichoke hearts, canned

½ cup sun-dried tomatoes (packed in water)

2 cups romaine lettuce

1 tablespoon Herb Vinaigrette Dressing (see recipe on page 163)

1 tablespoon walnuts, toasted and chopped

Mix artichoke hearts and tomatoes, and place over romaine. Top with dressing and walnuts.

MAKES 1 SERVING 362 CALORIES

Black Bean Tortillas with Pico de Gallo

¼ cup black beans, rinsed and drained

½ cup instant brown rice, cooked

¼ avocado, sliced

¼ cup Pico de Gallo (see recipe on page 166)

1 whole-grain tortilla (6-inch size)

Sea salt

Arrange black beans, brown rice, avocado slices and Pico de Gallo on a whole-grain tortilla. Add sea salt to taste. Roll up tortilla before eating.

MAKES 1 SERVING 351 CALORIES

Avocado Sandwich

1 teaspoon Dijon mustard

2 slices whole-grain bread, toasted

½ avocado, sliced

Sea salt

Pepper

½ tomato, sliced

½ cup alfalfa sprouts

3 romaine lettuce leaves

Spread Dijon mustard on one slice of toasted bread and place avocado on top. Sprinkle with salt and pepper to taste. Top with tomato, alfalfa sprouts, romaine and other slice of bread.

MAKES 1 SERVING 320 CALORIES

Instant Rice: A Huge Time-Saver

Instant brown and wild rice are two of my favorite staples. Mix up a batch of 2 or 3 cups, following package directions, and store in a container to add to lunches!

Simple Greek Salad

3 cups chopped romaine lettuce

½ small red onion, thinly sliced

¼ cup pitted black olives, canned

½ green bell pepper, chopped

½ red bell pepper, chopped

1 tomato, chopped

½ cucumber, sliced

2 tablespoons pine nuts

1 tablespoon Greek Salad Dressing (see recipe on page 162)

Combine first 8 ingredients in a large salad bowl. Top with dressing.

MAKES 1 SERVING 401 CALORIES

Tex-Mex Salad

3 cups mixed greens

½ cup black beans

½ cup corn

¼ cup onion, minced

½ cup tomato, chopped

3 tablespoons pine nuts

1 tablespoon Cilantro-Lime Dressing
(see recipe on page 163)

In a medium bowl, toss greens, beans, corn, onion, tomato and pine nuts. Top with dressing.

MAKES 1 SERVING 345 CALORIES

Thai Lettuce Wrap

4 romaine leaves

½ cucumber, cut lengthwise

1 carrot, shredded

½ tomato, chopped

½ cup bean sprouts

1 whole-grain tortilla (6-inch size)

1 tablespoon peanuts

1 tablespoon Peanut Dressing
(see recipe on page 162)

Place vegetables in a whole-grain tortilla. Add peanuts. Top with dressing. Roll up tortilla before eating.

MAKES 1 SERVING 345 CALORIES

Smashed White Bean and Avocado Sandwich

½ cup white beans

¼ of an avocado

1 teaspoon extra-virgin olive oil

Squeeze of lemon

Sea salt

Pepper

2 pieces whole-grain bread, toasted

2 slices red onion

¼ cucumber, sliced

3 pieces romaine lettuce

Combine the beans, avocado, olive oil and lemon in a medium bowl. Roughly mash the mixture until it comes together but is still a little chunky. Season with salt and pepper to taste. Spread the bean mixture on one slice of toasted bread. Top with red onion, cucumber slices and romaine. Add more salt and pepper to taste. Top with the other slice of bread.

MAKES 1 SERVING 333 CALORIES

Lettuce and Tomato Sandwich on a Bagel

Sea salt

1 beefsteak tomato, sliced thick

3 leaves romaine lettuce

1 teaspoon balsamic vinegar

1 whole-grain bagel, toasted or grilled

2 slices red onion

1 tablespoon Dijon mustard

Pepper

Sprinkle salt to taste on beefsteak tomato slices. Toss romaine and balsamic vinegar, and place on one half of toasted bagel. Top with a slice of red onion, and add more salt to taste.

Top lettuce and onion with tomato slices, and add mustard. Season with pepper to taste. Top with the other bagel half.

MAKES 1 SERVING 320 CALORIES

Potato Wrap

1 small potato, diced

1 teaspoon extra-virgin olive oil

Sea salt

Pepper

½ cup refried beans

Pinch of red pepper flakes

1 whole-grain tortilla (6-inch size)

½ avocado

1 cup baby spinach

Preheat oven to 425°F.

Place potato pieces on a baking sheet. Baste with olive oil, salt and pepper. Roast in the oven for about 15 minutes, until tender. Heat beans and red pepper flakes in microwave for 30 seconds and spread on tortilla. Top with potatoes, avocado and spinach. Roll up tortilla before eating.

MAKES 1 SERVING 370 CALORIES

Cold Quinoa Salad

1 cup broccoli, chopped

¼ cup red onion, finely chopped

½ cup tomato, chopped

½ cup sliced black olives

1 cup quinoa, cooked and chilled

1 tablespoon Herb Vinaigrette Dressing (see recipe on page 163)

1 tablespoon sunflower seeds

In a medium bowl, mix broccoli, onion, tomato and olives with quinoa. Top with dressing and sunflower seeds.

MAKES 1 SERVING 397 CALORIES

Tex-Mex Wrap

½ cup black beans

¼ cup corn

½ cup brown rice

1 whole-grain tortilla (6-inch size)

½ cup Pico de Gallo (store-bought or homemade; see recipe on page 166)

1 tablespoon pine nuts, toasted

Sriracha or other hot sauce

Mix black beans, corn and rice together. Place on tortilla. Top with Pico de Gallo and pine nuts, and add a dash of sriracha sauce. Roll up tortilla before eating.

MAKES 1 SERVING 325 CALORIES

Asian-Inspired Salad

3 cups mixed greens

½ cup green onion, minced

½ cup sliced red pepper

1 mandarin orange, peeled and separated

3 tablespoons almonds, slivered or crushed

1 tablespoon Asian Salad Dressing (see recipe on page 163)

10 Garlic Croutons (see recipe on page 164)

In a medium bowl, mix greens, onion, red pepper, mandarin orange and almonds. Top salad with dressing and croutons.

MAKES 1 SERVING 304 CALORIES

Brown Rice and Chickpea Salad (chilled)

½ cup instant brown rice, cooked

¼ cup chickpeas, rinsed and drained

½ cup canned pineapple in unsweetened juice (drain juice and reserve)

½ cup green onion, chopped

½ cup orange sections

1 tablespoon Lemon-Paprika Dressing (see recipe on page 163)

1 tablespoon pine nuts

In a large bowl, combine rice, chickpeas, pineapple, green onion and oranges. Top with dressing and pine nuts and toss gently to combine.

MAKES 1 SERVING 412 CALORIES

MIDAFTERNOON SNACK OPTIONS

Between lunch and dinner, you'll choose another snack from the list on pages 155–160. This will help keep you powered through afternoon until dinner.

DINNER OPTIONS

Most of us look forward to our evening meal as the reward after a hectic day, a chance to finally relax and unwind. These recipes are all quick and easy, yet will give your body's cells the "reboot" they need. **You have 21 choices** but, as before, choose seven different dinners to give your body the widest selection of nutrients. Each recipe makes three to four servings, so you'll have plenty to share with the family, or save for leftovers the next day.

Potato and Veggie Skillet

16 small new potatoes, sliced thick, skin left on

2 tablespoons extra-virgin olive oil, divided

3 carrots, chopped

3 medium zucchinis, chopped

3 medium yellow squash

4 teaspoons sea salt

4 teaspoons pepper

4 teaspoons red pepper flakes

In a large skillet, sauté potatoes in 1 tablespoon of olive oil, turning every few minutes, for 10 minutes. Steam additional vegetables until tender while potatoes are cooking. Toss steamed vegetables in with potatoes and remaining tablespoon of olive oil and flash-sauté. Season with salt, pepper and red pepper flakes.

MAKES 4 SERVINGS
420 CALORIES EACH

Broccoli and Wild Rice

8 cups broccoli florets

4 cups instant wild rice, cooked with vegetable broth instead of water

2 small onions, chopped

4 teaspoons garlic, minced

4 teaspoons extra-virgin olive oil

4 teaspoons cilantro

8 tablespoons pine nuts, toasted

In a large saucepan, steam broccoli until fork-tender. As broccoli cooks, prepare wild rice and set aside, covered, to keep warm.

In a small sauté pan, sauté onions and garlic in olive oil until soft. In a bowl, combine steamed broccoli, prepared rice, and onion and garlic mixture, tossing all ingredients together. Top with cilantro and pine nuts.

MAKES 4 SERVINGS
407 CALORIES EACH

Sweet Pea Pasta with Olive Oil

4 cups whole-grain pasta

2 cups frozen peas, thawed or steamed

2 tablespoons extra-virgin olive oil

Sea salt

Pepper

For side:

4 cups spinach, stems removed

1 tablespoon extra-virgin olive oil

1 tablespoon lemon juice

Cook pasta according to package directions. After draining the pasta, return it to the pot, and stir in thawed peas until heated through. Add olive oil and stir well. Add salt and pepper to taste.

For side: While pasta is cooking, in a large skillet, sauté spinach in olive oil until tender. Drizzle with lemon juice before serving.

MAKES 4 SERVINGS OF ABOUT 1 ½ CUPS PASTA AND 1 CUP SPINACH EACH 402 CALORIES EACH

Portabella Burger and Grilled Asparagus

1 tablespoon extra-virgin olive oil

2 tablespoons garlic, minced

4 tablespoons balsamic vinegar

4 large portabella mushrooms

8 slices whole-grain bread

1 tomato, sliced

4 slices onion

8 romaine lettuce leaves

For side:

16 large asparagus spears

1 tablespoon extra-virgin olive oil

Mix together olive oil, garlic and balsamic vinegar as a marinade. Grill mushrooms while basting with marinade for about 10 minutes; grill asparagus at the same time. Place mushrooms on whole-grain bread and top with tomato, onion, romaine and another slice of bread.

For side: Drizzle olive oil over grilled asparagus and serve.

MAKES 4 SERVINGS OF 1 PORTBELLA BURGER AND 4 SPEARS OF ASPARAGUS EACH 446 CALORIES EACH

Indonesian Peanut Rice

4 cups instant brown rice, cooked in vegetable broth

2 cups bean sprouts

1 medium red pepper, diced

1 cup cauliflower, chopped

2 cups watercress, chopped

¼ cup peanuts, roasted and chopped

For sauce:

3 tablespoons vinegar

3 tablespoons low-sodium soy sauce

¼ cup natural peanut butter

½ tablespoon red pepper flakes

Cook brown rice according to package directions; set aside in pot. In a steamer, cook vegetables until tender.

For sauce: Mix vinegar, soy sauce, peanut butter and red pepper flakes in a saucepan over medium heat and cook until peanut butter is melted and ingredients are well blended.

Toss the veggies with the sauce and rice, and top with peanuts.

MAKES 4 SERVINGS OF ABOUT 2 CUPS EACH 430 CALORIES EACH

Cuban-Style Rice and Beans with Mango

1 ¼ cups onion, chopped

1 ¼ cups green bell pepper, chopped

1 tablespoon garlic, minced

½ teaspoon cumin

½ tomato, chopped

1 tablespoon extra-virgin olive oil

1 teaspoon sea salt

1 teaspoon hot pepper sauce

½ teaspoon thyme

1 fifteen-ounce can kidney beans, rinsed and drained with liquid reserved

1 medium mango, diced

4 cups brown rice, cooked

Sauté onion, pepper, garlic, cumin and tomato in olive oil over medium heat, adding salt, pepper sauce and thyme, until veggies are tender.

Stir in beans, reserved liquid and mango and cook until warmed through.

Serve over rice.

**MAKES 4 SERVINGS OF ABOUT ¾ CUP EACH, WITH 1 CUP RICE
383 CALORIES EACH**

Spinach and Bean Casserole

1 medium onion, chopped

1 tablespoon garlic, minced

2 carrots, chopped

2 celery stalks, chopped

2 cups spinach, washed and chopped

1 teaspoon sea salt

1 tablespoon extra-virgin olive oil

4 cups white beans

Preheat oven to 350°F.

Sauté onion, garlic, carrots, celery, spinach and salt in olive oil until soft, about 15 minutes. Add white beans and pour into a medium-sized casserole dish. Bake for 15 minutes and slice into quarters to serve.

**MAKES 4 SERVINGS
398 CALORIES EACH**

Brussels Sprouts Ragout

8 whole shallots

4 tablespoons extra-virgin olive oil

6 cups Brussels sprouts, halved

4 carrots, sliced into coin-sized pieces

3 cups navy beans

2 cups vegetable broth

2 tablespoons garlic, minced

Preheat oven to 500°F.

Slice the root end off shallots and toss them in oil. Wrap in foil and roast in the oven until tender. While the shallots are roasting, steam the Brussels sprouts and carrots until tender, about 8–10 minutes.

Slip roasted shallots from skin. In a large pan, add navy beans, vegetable broth, garlic and vegetables to shallots, gently stirring to coat.

**MAKES 4 SERVINGS
377 CALORIES EACH**

Quinoa with Sun-Dried Tomatoes

4 cups quinoa, cooked

½ cup sun-dried tomatoes, packed in water, drained and chopped

¼ cup extra-virgin olive oil

¼ cup balsamic vinegar

½ cup pine nuts, toasted

1 tablespoon garlic, minced

Cook quinoa according to package directions. Drain well and add tomatoes, olive oil, vinegar, pine nuts and garlic. Let cool before serving.

**MAKES 4 SERVINGS
427 CALORIES EACH**

Wild Rice Skillet

4 cups baby kale

1 small onion, diced

1 tablespoon extra-virgin olive oil

4 cups butternut squash, diced

1 teaspoon dried thyme

2 tablespoons balsamic vinegar

2 cups wild rice, cooked

In a skillet, sauté kale and onion with olive oil and set aside, covered to keep warm. Steam butternut squash for 10 minutes or until tender.

Toss steamed squash in skillet with kale mixture and flash-cook for five minutes, adding thyme and balsamic vinegar before serving over wild rice.

**MAKES 4 SERVINGS
415 CALORIES EACH**

Pasta Primavera

4 cups whole-grain pasta

1 tablespoon extra-virgin olive oil

1 cup red bell pepper, chopped

3 cups broccoli florets

1 zucchini, cut into 1-inch slices

1 teaspoon sea salt

2 teaspoons garlic, minced

½ cup fresh basil, finely chopped

Pepper

Cook pasta according to package directions.

While pasta is cooking, in a sauté pan, heat olive oil over medium-high heat. Sauté pepper, broccoli and zucchini with salt and garlic until fork-tender. Divide vegetables over 1 cup of cooked pasta per serving and top each plate with fresh basil, salt and pepper.

**MAKES 4 SERVINGS OF ABOUT
2 CUPS EACH 402 CALORIES EACH**

Veggie Fajitas

1 red pepper, sliced

1 yellow pepper, sliced

2 small yellow onions, sliced

2 cups mushrooms, sliced

1 tablespoon extra-virgin olive oil

2 cups black beans

4 corn tortillas (6-inch size)

2 cups lettuce

2 cups tomatoes, chopped

1 avocado, cored, peeled and sliced

2 cups brown rice, cooked

In a sauté pan, sauté sliced peppers, onions and mushrooms in olive oil. Add black beans and warm.

Assemble fajitas by placing bean mixture on tortillas; add lettuce, tomatoes and avocado. Serve with rice.

MAKES 4 SERVINGS
407 CALORIES EACH

Penne with Tomatoes and Kale

4 cups whole-grain penne

2 cups kale

1 tablespoon garlic, minced

1 tablespoon extra-virgin olive oil

2 cups tomato, chopped

Sea salt

Pepper

Fresh parsley

Cook pasta according to package directions.

While pasta is cooking, in a large sauté pan over medium-high heat, sauté kale and garlic in olive oil for about 5 minutes or until it begins to wilt. Add tomato and cooked pasta and continue to sauté, stirring gently to combine, until heated through. Add salt and pepper to taste. Serve with fresh parsley.

MAKES 4 SERVINGS
400 CALORIES EACH

Vegan Chili

2 tablespoons extra-virgin olive oil

1 large onion, diced

1 tablespoon garlic, minced

3 stalks celery, chopped

2 red peppers, diced

2 large tomatoes, diced

1 cup water

2 cups red kidney beans

1 cup black beans

1 cup frozen corn

1 teaspoon oregano

1 tablespoon chili powder

Sea salt

Pepper

Heat oil in a large pot over medium-high heat. Add onion, garlic, celery, peppers and tomatoes to pan and sauté for about 10 minutes. Add water, kidney beans, black beans and corn, plus oregano, chili powder and 1 teaspoon salt. Let the chili return to a simmer. Cook for 5 minutes or until the corn and beans are heated through. Generously salt and pepper to taste.

MAKES 4 SERVINGS
395 CALORIES EACH

Black Bean-Topped Sweet Potatoes

4 medium sweet potatoes

2 tablespoons extra-virgin olive oil

2 tablespoons garlic, minced

1 cup onion, chopped

1 cup green pepper, chopped

4 cups black beans, cooked

2 cups fresh salsa

4 teaspoons cumin

2 teaspoons sea salt

1 teaspoon black pepper

Preheat oven to 400°F.

Pierce sweet potatoes with a fork several times, then place them directly on the oven rack. Bake for 45 minutes, or until fork-tender. While potatoes are cooling, prepare the bean filling.

Heat the oil in a large sauté pan over medium-high heat. Sauté garlic, onion and pepper until soft. Stir in the black beans, salsa and seasonings. Cook until heated through. When potatoes are cool, cut each in half lengthwise and top with the bean filling.

MAKES 4 SERVINGS
423 CALORIES EACH

Spinach and Artichoke Pasta Bake

12 cups baby spinach

2 cups canned artichoke hearts, in water

1 tablespoon garlic, minced

4 cups tomatoes, chopped

2 tablespoons extra-virgin olive oil

3 cups vegetable broth

4 cups whole-grain pasta, cooked

2 cups Garlic Croutons (see recipe on page 164), crushed

Preheat oven to 350°F.

In a small bowl, combine spinach, artichoke hearts, garlic, tomatoes, olive oil and broth to make all ingredients wet and incorporated. Place cooked pasta in the bottom of a medium-sized casserole dish. Top with the spinach mixture. Top that with the crushed croutons and bake 20 minutes. Cut into quarters and serve.

MAKES 4 SERVINGS
400 CALORIES EACH

Pepper and Cauliflower Hash

8 cups cauliflower florets

4 medium zucchini, sliced

5 teaspoons garlic, minced

4 cups red peppers, roasted and packed in water

4 teaspoons extra-virgin olive oil

2 teaspoons sea salt

1 teaspoon pepper

2 cups fresh basil, chopped

4 tablespoons pine nuts, roasted

In a large sauté pan, sauté cauliflower, zucchini, garlic and peppers in olive oil for 15 minutes, or until vegetables are tender. Season with salt and pepper; add basil and pine nuts.

MAKES 4 SERVINGS
393 CALORIES EACH

Cream of Broccoli and Pistachio Soup

1 small onion, diced

4 teaspoons garlic, minced

8 cups broccoli florets

2 cups pistachios, shelled and chopped

2 tablespoons extra-virgin olive oil

6 cups vegetable broth

2 cups unsweetened almond milk

1 teaspoon cayenne pepper

Squeeze of lemon juice

In a large saucepan, sauté onion, garlic, broccoli and pistachios in olive oil for a few minutes. Add vegetable broth and simmer until broccoli is tender. Transfer ingredients in batches to a blender and blend until smooth. Return soup to the pan. Add the almond milk to the pan. Stir in the cayenne pepper and lemon juice until heated through.

**MAKES 4 SERVINGS
335 CALORIES EACH**

Stuffed Peppers

2 cups lentils, cooked

2 zucchini, chopped

2 small yellow onions, diced small

1 tablespoon garlic, minced

2 carrots, diced small

2 jalapeño peppers, diced small

2 tablespoons extra-virgin olive oil

4 red bell peppers

2 teaspoons fresh basil, chopped

2 cups bean sprouts

2 teaspoons cayenne pepper

½ cup sunflower seeds

Preheat oven to 400°F.

Cook lentils according to package directions and set aside. In a large sauté pan, sauté zucchini, onions, garlic, carrots and jalapeño peppers in olive oil until onions are soft. As mixture cooks, core the red peppers and place them in a casserole dish. Fill the peppers with the lentils and vegetable mixture. Add a half inch of water to the pan and bake for 20 minutes.

Add basil, sprouts and cayenne pepper to the peppers, and heat until just warmed through; add sunflower seeds on top.

**MAKES 4 SERVINGS (EACH PEPPER IS ONE SERVING)
395 CALORIES EACH**

Veggie Couscous

2 cups couscous, cooked

8 cups vegetable broth

1 onion, chopped

2 cups mushrooms, sliced

2 teaspoons garlic, minced

2 tablespoons extra-virgin olive oil

4 tablespoons lemon juice

4 teaspoons oregano

4 cups fresh spinach, coarsely chopped

1 cup pine nuts

In a saucepan, combine the couscous and broth over medium heat.

In a separate skillet, sauté the onion, mushrooms and garlic in olive oil until tender. Stir in the lemon juice and oregano. Add spinach, cooking only until wilted.

Toss the cooked couscous with the spinach mixture and top with pine nuts.

MAKES 4 SERVINGS
402 CALORIES EACH

Veggie Soup

10 cups vegetable broth

4 cups frozen spinach

4 cups frozen corn

6 tomatoes, chopped

2 cups white beans

2 tablespoons rosemary

1 teaspoon sea salt

1 teaspoon pepper

2 teaspoons garlic powder

Place all ingredients in a medium-sized pot and bring to a boil. Reduce heat and simmer for 30 minutes.

MAKES 4 SERVINGS
420 CALORIES EACH

So now you've seen all the recipes and the "base" version of all the wonderful cleansing foods that you will be using in this program. (In Phase 2 and thereafter, you'll include additional protein to the lunches and dinners.)

There is so much selection to choose from, you should never get bored! I know it's easy to eat the same favorites every day, but challenge yourself and try all of them through the 21-day program. Each meal has different nutrients that will change your body chemistry, so think of yourself as a scientist and not just a chef. Have fun tasting new flavors—I know I did as I created this menu!

MENU PLAN

Here is a sample menu plan for Phase 1 (that is, week 1) on the detox plan:

MONDAY (DAY 1)

Breakfast: Grape-Lime Smoothie (see recipe on page 151)

Snack: Almond Butter and Celery (see recipe on page 156)

Lunch: Chopped Italian Salad (see recipe on page 165)

Snack: Bell Peppers with Sweet Potato Hummus (see recipe on page 158)

Dinner: Indonesian Peanut Rice (see recipe on page 174)

After Dinner: Ginger Detox Tea (see recipe on page 147)

TUESDAY (DAY 2)

Breakfast: Mango-Strawberry Smoothie (see recipe on page 152)

Snack: Spicy Avocado (see recipe on page 159)

Lunch: Brown Rice and Chickpea Salad (see recipe on page 171)

Snack: Spicy Toasted Chickpeas (see recipe on page 157)

Dinner: Black Bean-Topped Sweet Potatoes (see recipe on page 179)

After Dinner: Ginger Detox Tea (see recipe on page 147)

WEDNESDAY (DAY 3)

Breakfast: Carrot-Orange Smoothie (see recipe on page 152)

Snack: Cinnamon-Apple Slices (see recipe on page 159)

Lunch: Tex-Mex Wrap (see recipe on page 171)

Snack: Guacamole and Chips (see recipe on page 160)

Dinner: Veggie Soup (see recipe on page 182)

After Dinner: Ginger Detox Tea (see recipe on page 147)

THURSDAY (DAY 4)

Breakfast: Super Spinach Smoothie (see recipe on page 154)

Snack: Coconut Pineapple (see recipe on page 158)

Lunch: Simple Greek Salad (see recipe on page 168)

Snack: Frozen Grapes with Pumpkin Seeds (see recipe on page 159)

Dinner: Cuban-Style Rice and Beans with Mango (see recipe on page 175)

After Dinner: Ginger Detox Tea (see recipe on page 147)

FRIDAY (DAY 5)

Breakfast: Cran-Blueberry Smoothie (see recipe on page 153)

Snack: Honey Pear (see recipe on page 158)

Lunch: Avocado Sandwich (see recipe on page 168)

Snack: Almond-Kale Chips (see recipe on page 158)

Dinner: Portabella Burger and Grilled Asparagus (see recipe on page 174)

After Dinner: Ginger Detox Tea (see recipe on page 147)

SATURDAY (DAY 6)

Breakfast: Super-Antioxidant Smoothie (see recipe on page 152)

Snack: Quick Wrap (see recipe on page 159)

Lunch: Lettuce and Tomato Sandwich on a Bagel (see recipe on page 170)

Snack: Artichoke Dip and Carrots (see recipe on page 160)

Dinner: Quinoa with Sun-Dried Tomatoes (see recipe on page 176)

After Dinner: Ginger Detox Tea (see recipe on page 147)

SUNDAY (DAY 7)

Breakfast: Pineapple-Mixed Berry Smoothie (see recipe on page 151)

Snack: Carrots/Celery and Hummus (see recipe on page 155)

Lunch: Pear and Bell Pepper Salad (see recipe on page 167)

Snack: Tomato with Pine Nuts (see recipe on page 156)

Dinner: Pasta Primavera (see recipe on page 177)

After Dinner: Ginger Detox Tea (see recipe on page 147)

THE PRIME WORKOUT

The prime workout is designed to teach you the basic movements you need to incorporate for a lifetime. The workout should take only about 20 minutes a day.

Each day, you'll perform four exercises that mainly target two muscle groups. After doing each set of four exercises, rest for one minute and then move to the next set. Doing more than one exercise in a row without rest is called a "superset" and increases the demand on your muscles as well as your heart. While this workout is simple to perform, doing supersets will keep your heart rate high, boosting cardiovascular health, and help "prime" your muscles for the challenging, new methods of training that come in the next two weeks.

I've suggested starting weights for women and men; your intensity level should be high enough that the last five reps are challenging. You may feel as if the muscles you're working are burning or growing fatigued during those reps. That means you're nearing muscle failure, where you're unable to perform another rep. Muscle failure on the last rep is exactly where you want to be.

Pay close attention to the description of the movements and follow the photos. If you can't perform a move with good form, choose lighter dumbbells. If you can complete a set with good form, increase your weights. Also, increase your weights every four weeks to continue to challenge your body. You'll need a couple of pairs of dumbbells for these moves. Use the heavier weights for your primary muscle groups (legs, chest and back) and lighter weights for your secondary muscle groups (shoulders, biceps and triceps).

Suggested Weights (If You Don't Exercise Regularly):

	Primary	Secondary
Women	15-lb dumbbells	8-lb dumbbells
Men	25-lb dumbbells	15-lb dumbbells

Suggested Weights (For Regular Exercisers):

	Primary	Secondary
Women	25-lb dumbbells	15-lb dumbbells
Men	40-lb dumbbells	20-lb dumbbells

Each day, you'll do four sets of four different exercises for 10 reps each. Don't worry, these are easy movements that will be the template for all the fun workouts to come. The schedule is specified below; the exercise descriptions follow that. You'll work all the major muscle groups (those in your legs, back and chest) and your core—the muscles in your abdomen—which you're already working doing these moves. Remember to run through all four exercises with little or no rest to equal one set then repeat three more times.

Phase 1 Workout: PRIME

PRIMARY	SECONDARY
MONDAY (or Day 1: Chest/Biceps)	
Flat Dumbbell Press: 10 reps/4 sets	Close Curl: 10 reps/4 sets
Flat Dumbbell Fly: 10 reps/4 sets	Hammer Curl: 10 reps/4 sets
TUESDAY (or Day 2: Back/Triceps)	
Wide Row: 10 reps/4 sets	Standing Alternating Tricep Extension: 10 reps/4 sets
Alternating Row: 10 reps/4 sets	Lying Down Head-Banger: 10 reps/4 sets
WEDNESDAY (or Day 3: Legs/Shoulders)	
Squat: 10 reps/4 sets	WV: 10 reps/4 sets
Front Lunge: 10 reps/4 sets	Around-the-Worlds : 10 reps/4 sets
THURSDAY (or Day 4: Chest/Biceps)	
Hammer Chest Press: 10 reps/4 sets	Diagonal Curl: 10 reps/4 sets
Reverse Press: 10 reps/4 sets	Wide Curl: 10 reps/4 sets
FRIDAY (or Day 5: Back/Triceps)	
Bent Row: 10 reps/4 sets	Kickback: 10 reps/4 sets
Reverse Row: 10 reps/4 sets	Standing Head-Banger: 10 reps/4 sets
SATURDAY (or Day 6: Legs/Shoulders)	
Plié Squat: 10 reps/4 sets	Arnold Press: 10 reps/4 sets
Backward Lunge: 10 reps/4 sets	Lateral Raise: 10 reps/4 sets
SUNDAY (or Day 7: Rest Day)	

THE BASIC MOVES

Now, let's get started! Here are the basic bodybuilding movements you should memorize and use for a lifetime.

MONDAY

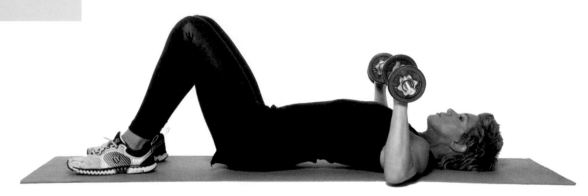

FLAT DUMBBELL PRESS

Lie on your back on a weight bench or the floor, dumbbells in both hands with your knuckles facing the ceiling, elbows making a 90-degree angle. Your feet should be together and your abs engaged (imagine pulling them back toward your spine). Engage your chest muscles and press the weights toward the ceiling before returning to the starting position.

10REPS X 4SETS

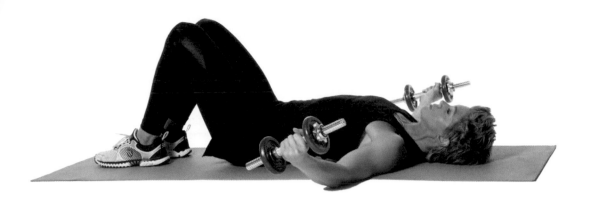

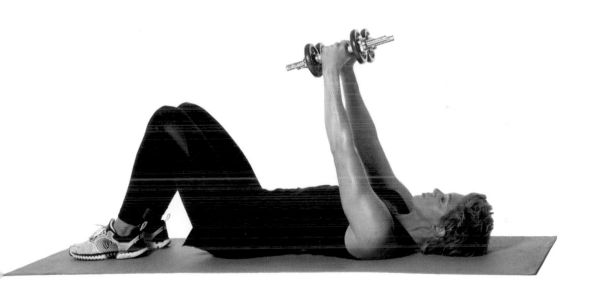

FLAT DUMBBELL FLY

Lie on your back, dumbbells in both hands with your arms wide
out and slightly bent. Your feet should be under your hips and your
abs engaged. Keeping your arms open, raise them over your chest
then return to the starting position.

10REPS X 4SETS

MONDAY
CONTINUED

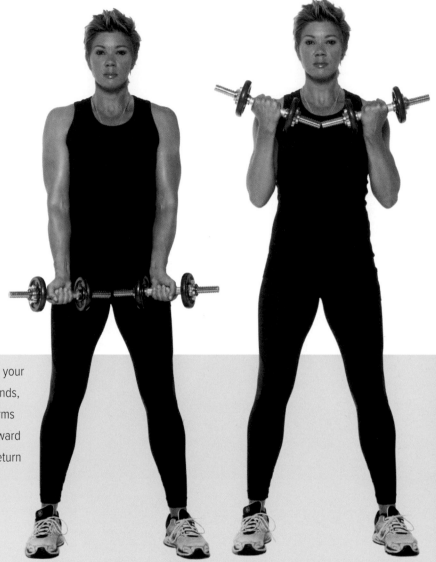

CLOSE CURL

Stand with your feet under your hips, dumbbells in both hands, arms in front. Bend your arms to bring the weights up toward your shoulders and then return to the starting position.

10REPS
X 4SETS

HAMMER CURL

Stand with your feet to the side of your hips, dumbbells in both hands, knuckles facing out. Bend your arms to bring the weights up toward your shoulders and then return to the starting position.

10REPS
X 4SETS

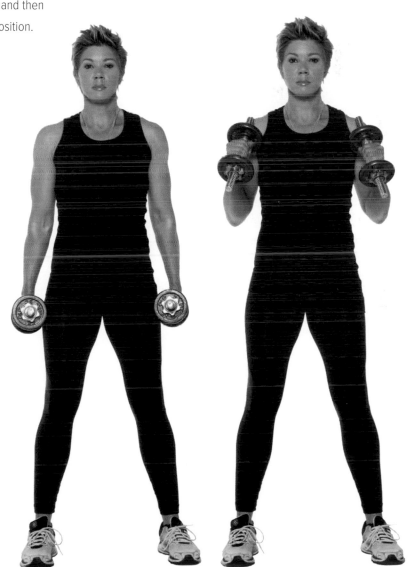

TUESDAY

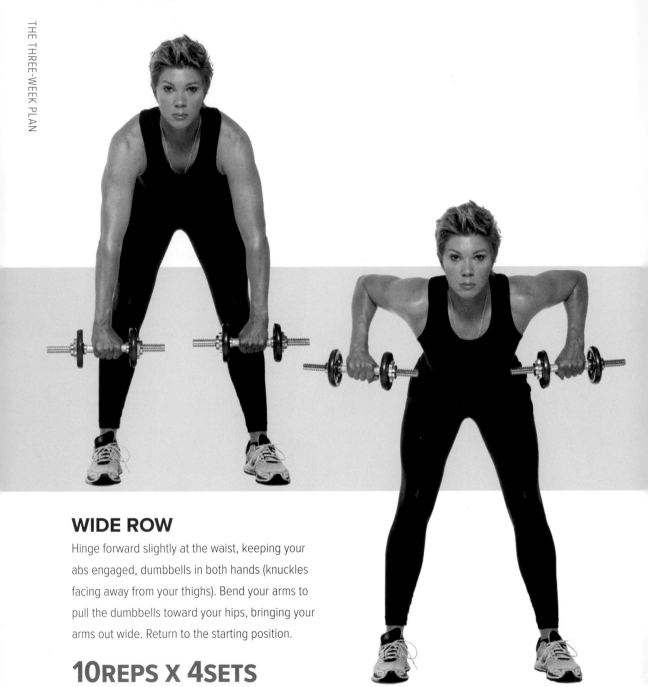

WIDE ROW

Hinge forward slightly at the waist, keeping your abs engaged, dumbbells in both hands (knuckles facing away from your thighs). Bend your arms to pull the dumbbells toward your hips, bringing your arms out wide. Return to the starting position.

10REPS X 4SETS

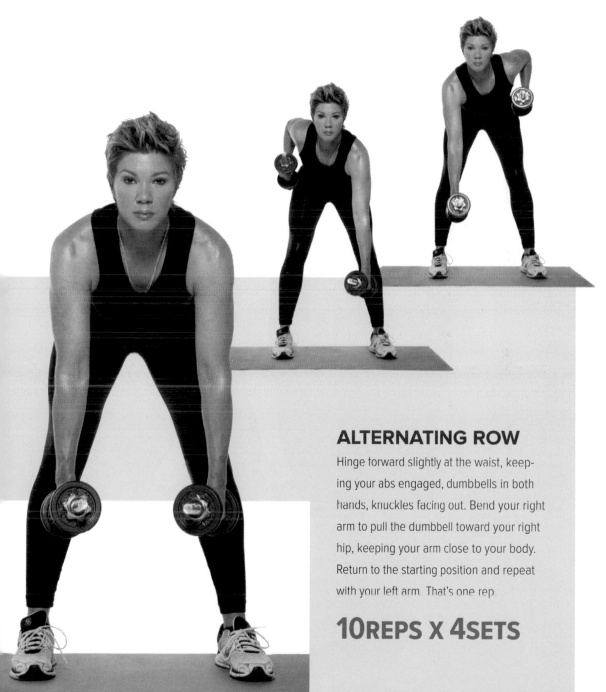

ALTERNATING ROW

Hinge forward slightly at the waist, keeping your abs engaged, dumbbells in both hands, knuckles facing out. Bend your right arm to pull the dumbbell toward your right hip, keeping your arm close to your body. Return to the starting position and repeat with your left arm. That's one rep.

10REPS X 4SETS

TUESDAY
CONTINUED

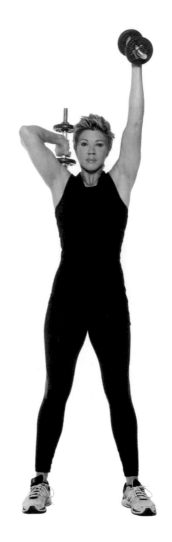

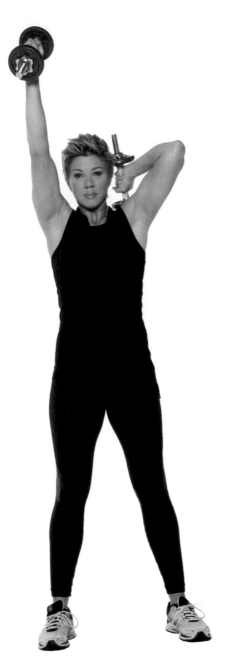

STANDING ALTERNATING TRICEP EXTENSION

Stand with your feet shoulder-width apart, dumbbells in both hands, knuckles facing out. Start with one arm fully extended to the ceiling, and the other forearm bent back behind your head. Alternate raising your forearm toward the ceiling as you lower the other forearm behind your head. That's one rep.

10REPS X 4SETS

LYING DOWN HEAD-BANGER

Lie on your back on a weight bench or the floor with your knees bent, and feet on the floor. Hold dumbbells in both hands with your knuckles facing the ceiling, arms over your shoulders. Brace your abs and bend your elbows to lower the dumbbells back toward your forehead (hence the name "head-bangers") before pressing back up to the starting position.

10REPS X 4SETS

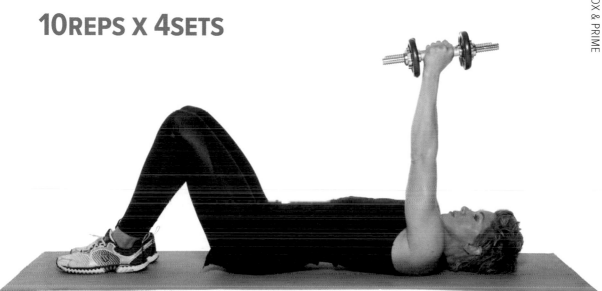

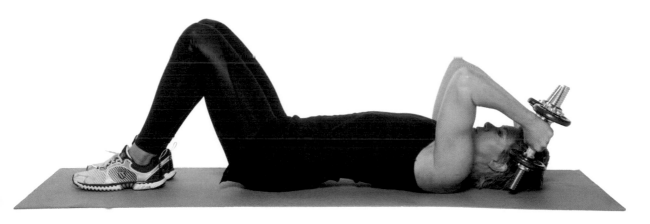

WEDNESDAY

SQUAT

Stand with your feet just slightly wider than hip-width apart, toes pointed slightly out, holding dumbbells in both hands. Engage your abdominal muscles and, keeping your chest up, bend your knees to push your bottom back and down as if you were going to sit on a bench or chair behind you. Lower your body until your thighs are parallel to the ground (or as low as feels comfortable to you) and return to the starting position.

10REPS
x 4SETS

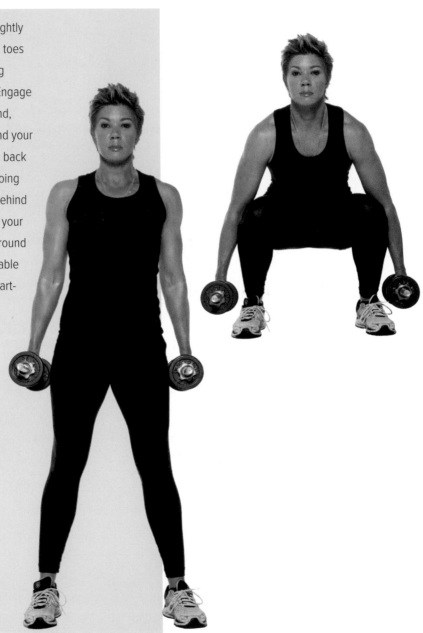

FRONT LUNGE

Stand with your feet directly under your hips, dumbbells in both hands. Step forward with your right leg, making a large enough step so that your right knee makes a 90-degree angle as you lower your left knee toward the ground. Then straighten your left leg and step back with your right leg to the starting position. Repeat, stepping forward with your left leg, lowering your right knee to the ground. That's one rep.

10REPS x 4SETS

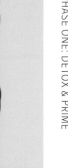

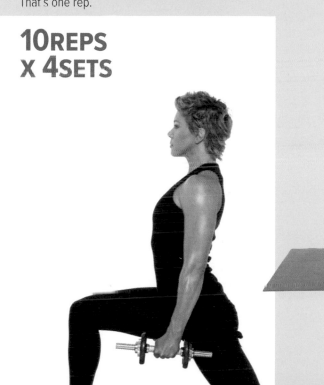

WEDNESDAY

CONTINUED

WV

Stand with your feet under your hips, dumbbells in both hands, arms bent and at your sides, knuckles facing out. (Your arms will form the letter "W.") Press the dumbbells up and out in a slight diagonal so that your arms are straight. Your arms now form the letter "V." Return to the starting position with arms bent by your sides.

10REPS X 4SETS

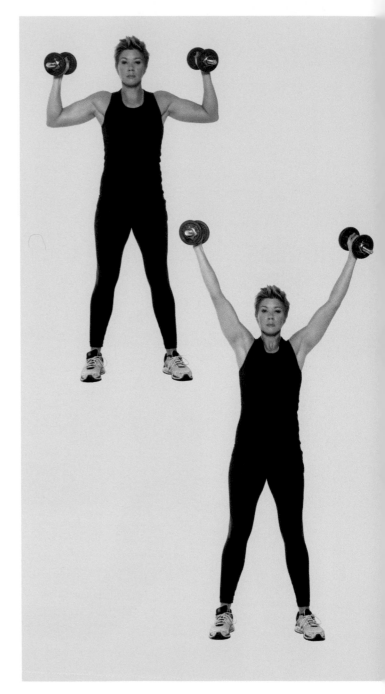

AROUND-THE-WORLD

Stand with your feet under your hips, hands in front, knuckles facing legs. Keeping your arms straight, slowly move the dumbbells upward in a circular motion above your head. Lower down following the same path. Each complete circle is one rep.

10REPS X 4SETS

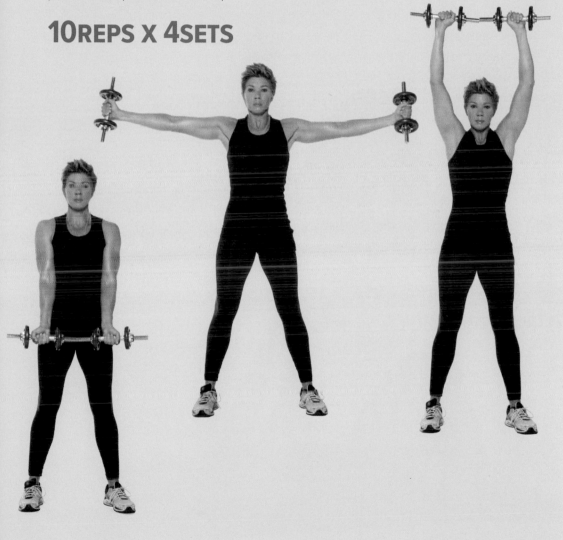

THURSDAY

HAMMER CHEST PRESS

Lie on your back on a weight bench or the floor with your knees bent, feet together, dumbbells in both hands with your knuckles facing out, elbows making a 90 degree angle. Engage your chest muscles and press the weights toward the ceiling before returning to the starting position.

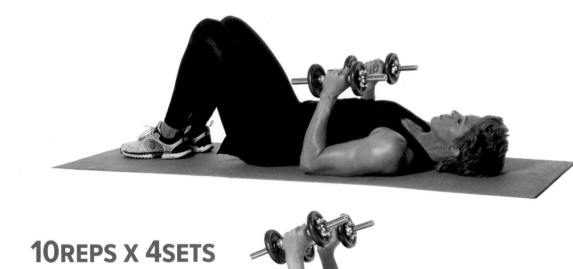

10REPS x 4SETS

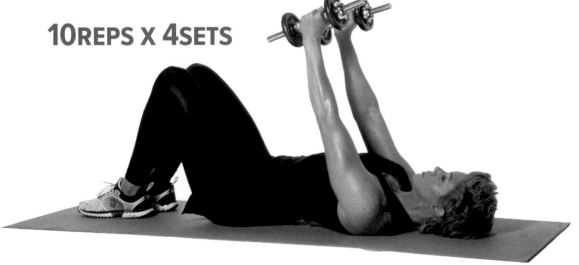

REVERSE PRESS

Lie on your back on a weight bench or the floor, dumbbells in both hands, and press up with your hands above your chest, knuckles facing out. Lower the dumbbells until your elbows make a 90-degree angle and then press up to the starting position.

10REPS x 4SETS

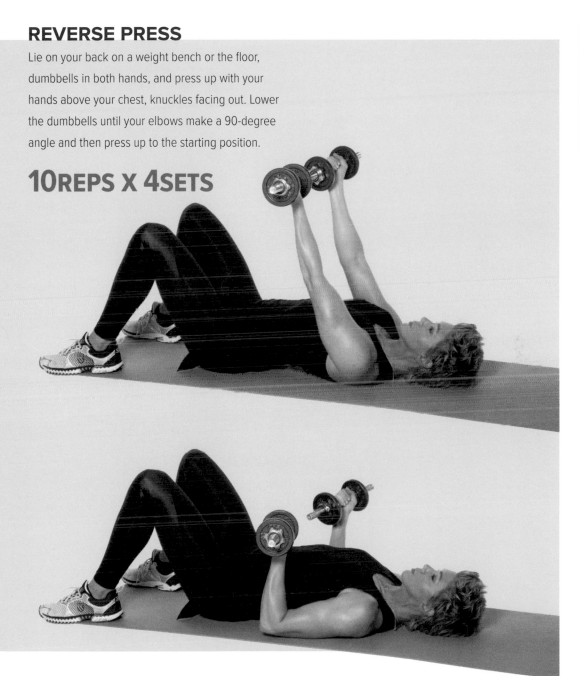

THURSDAY
CONTINUED

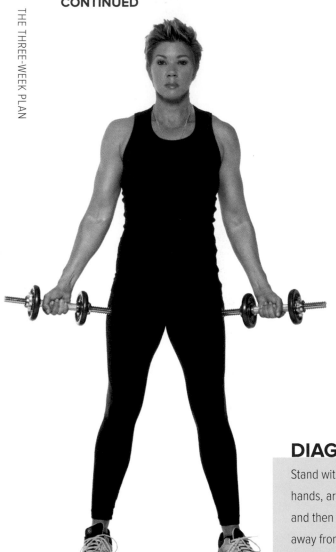

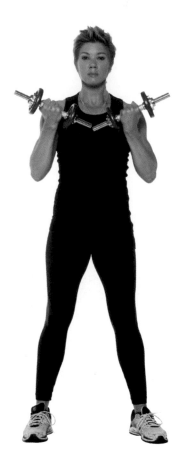

DIAGONAL CURL

Stand with your feet under your hips, dumbbells in both hands, arms at your natural carrying angle at your sides, and then move your hands about three inches farther away from your body. In a diagonal motion, curl your arms upward toward your chest. Return to the starting position.

10REPS x 4SETS

WIDE CURL

Stand with your feet under your hips, dumbbells in both hands, arms at your natural carrying angle at your sides, and then move your hands about three inches farther away from your body. Bend your arms to bring the weights up toward your shoulders and then return to the starting position.

10 REPS X 4 SETS

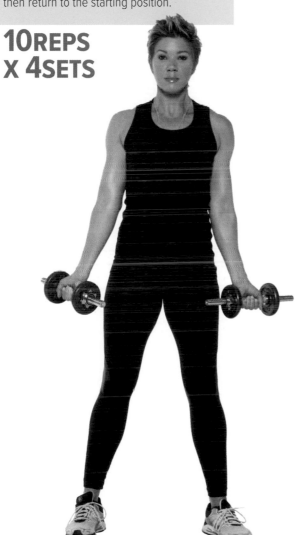
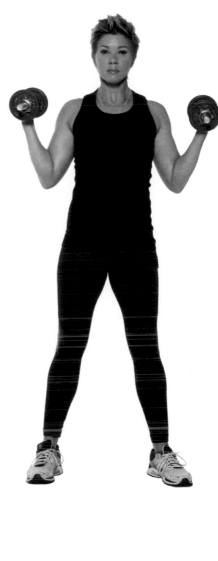

FRIDAY

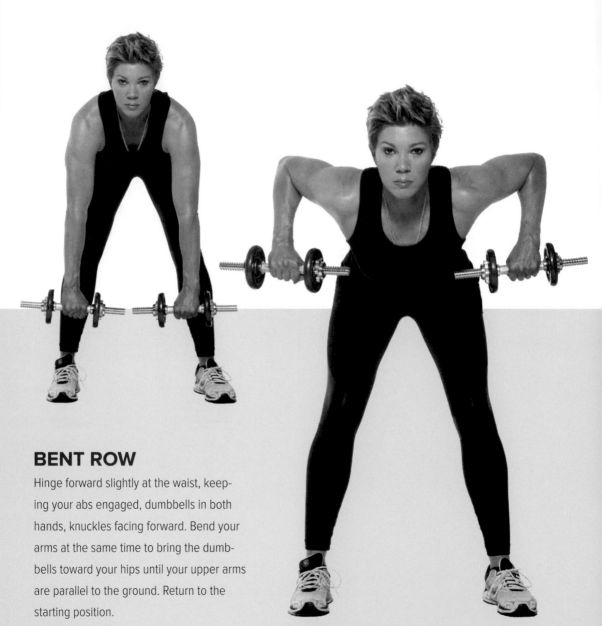

BENT ROW

Hinge forward slightly at the waist, keeping your abs engaged, dumbbells in both hands, knuckles facing forward. Bend your arms at the same time to bring the dumbbells toward your hips until your upper arms are parallel to the ground. Return to the starting position.

10REPS X 4SETS

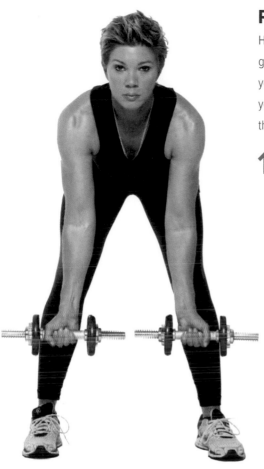

REVERSE ROW

Hinge forward slightly at the waist, keeping your abs engaged, dumbbells in both hands, with your knuckles facing your thighs. Bend your arms to pull the dumbbells toward your hips, keeping your arms close to your body. Return to the starting position.

10REPS X 4SETS

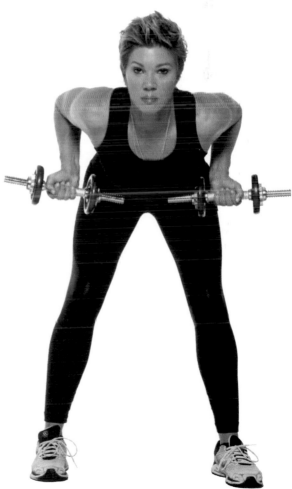

FRIDAY
CONTINUED

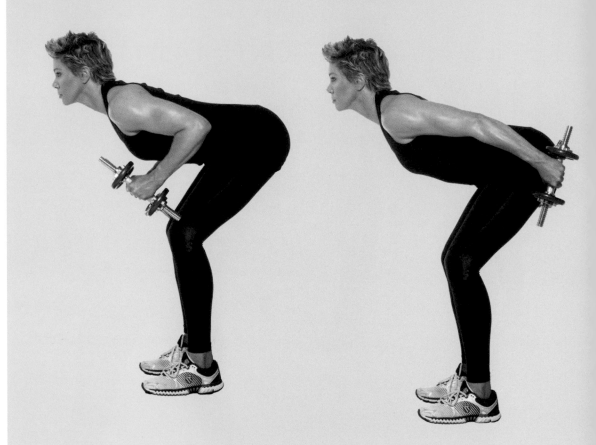

KICKBACK

Stand with feet shoulder-width apart and bend at the waist. Hold both dumbbells at a 90-degree angle, then straighten to align with your back. Return to starting position.

10REPS X 4SETS

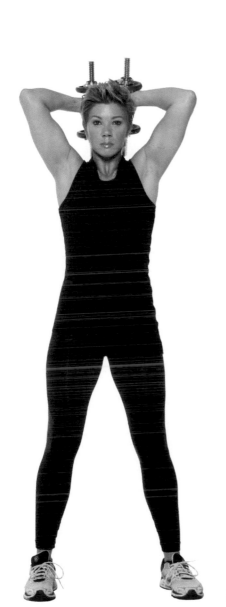
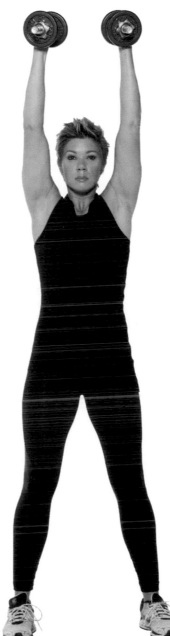

STANDING HEAD-BANGER

Stand with your feet under your hips, holding dumbbells in both hands behind your head. Keeping your upper arms close to your head, straighten your arms to raise the dumbbells over your head. Lower the dumbbells back to the starting position.

10REPS X 4SETS

SATURDAY

PLIÉ SQUAT

Stand with your feet wide apart (about a foot wider than your regular squat stance), toes pointed slightly out, holding one dumbbell in your hands. Engage your abdominal muscles. Keeping your chest up, bend your knees to push your bottom back and down as if you were going to sit on a bench or a chair behind you. Lower your body until your thighs are nearly parallel to the ground and return to the starting position.

10REPS X 4SETS

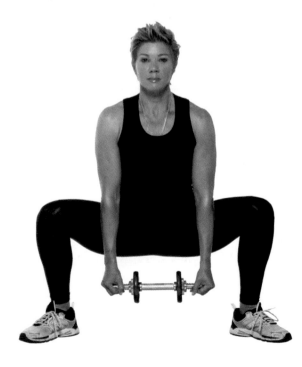

BACKWARD LUNGE

Stand with your feet directly under your hips, dumbbells in both hands. Step backward with your right leg, making a large enough step so that both your right knee and your left knee make a 90-degree angle. Step forward to a standing position. Repeat with left leg. That's one rep.

10REPS X 4SETS

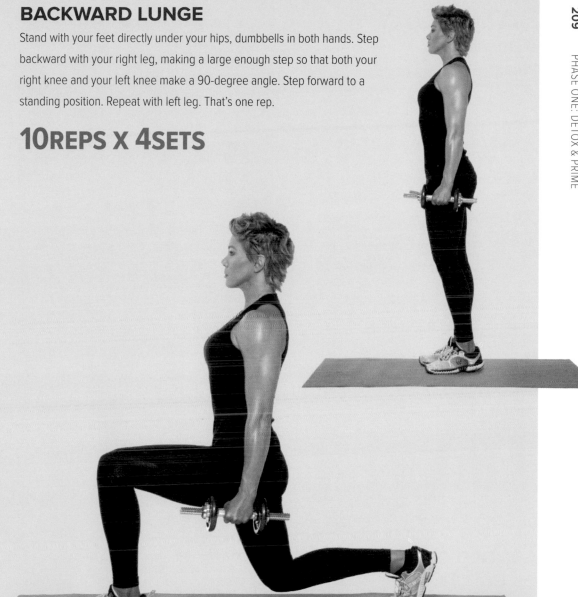

SATURDAY
CONTINUED

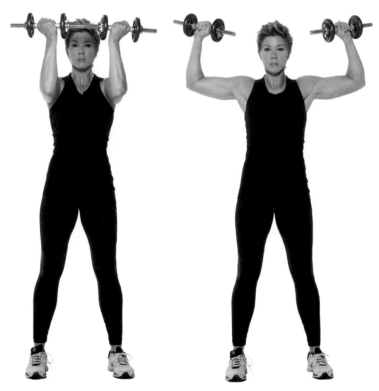

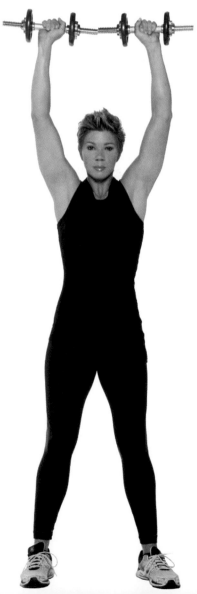

ARNOLD PRESS

Stand with your feet under your hips, dumbbells at shoulder height, in front of your face, knuckles facing out. Engage your abdominals and take your elbows out to the sides. Press the dumbbells over your head until your arms are straight. Return to the starting position.

10REPS X 4SETS

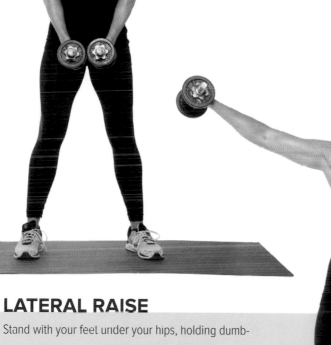

LATERAL RAISE

Stand with your feet under your hips, holding dumb-bells in both hands with your arms in front of your body. Engage your abdominals and, keeping your arms straight, raise them two inches above your shoulder height. Return to the starting position.

10REPS X 4SETS

CHAPTER EIGHT

PHASE TWO: BALANCE & BURN

Now that your cells are working at their best, it's time to focus on balance—balancing sleep cycles, hormones and insulin levels by introducing amino acids and spices. The workouts you'll do in this week are specialized for ultimate balance and fat-burning. When homeostasis, meaning stable state, is achieved, your metabolism, energy and mood will skyrocket. The body craves balance; these seven days in Phase 2 will help restore it.

THE BALANCE DIET (ANIMAL PROTEINS)

Last week, in Phase 1, you followed the detox diet, which was designed to cleanse and detoxify your body's cells and provide the essential nutrients they need to function optimally. Think of the detox diet as the "base" foods for the entire program. In each phase you will build upon that foundation to treat every aspect of what is making you sick and tired. This week, in Phase 2, we will add animal protein and spices that balance insulin levels and hormones with their powerful ingredients, creating maximum internal stability. The addition will promote steady energy and quality sleep by normalizing adrenal and thyroid functions, and create cleaner metabolic functions by accelerating glucose turnover and regulating insulin response.

Protein, which is made up of amino acids, is essential not only for building muscle, but also for weight loss. Consuming sufficient protein for your body's needs helps you lose weight if you need to, and contributes to sleek, strong muscles. While foods such as fruits, vegetables and grains contain amino acids, animal protein sources are considered "complete proteins," meaning that they contain all eight amino acids our bodies can't manufacture on their own.

Free Range— The Best!

I'm not playin'. I have already told you that factory-farmed meats are extremely toxic to you, causing you to be fat, sluggish and diseased. I use and refer everyone to this amazing site, www.localharvest.org. All you do is type in your zip code and it will guide you to free-range markets and restaurants and show you a list of local farmers so that you can start eating healthy. Almost all grocery stores around the nation have free-range meats and dairy—if my mom and family can eat free-range in my little Midwest hometown, so can you.

If you cannot find free-range meats, then *do not add meat and dairy* to the next seven days unless it is freshwater seafood. Simply add three-ounce servings of plant-based proteins such as black beans, chickpeas or quinoa to your lunches and dinners.

Foods this week will contain the highest amount of gland- and insulin-balancing ingredients, such as iodine, selenium, essential fatty acids, copper and iron. You're already consuming plenty of foods that contain vitamin C, which helps increase the absorption of nutrients. Last week, you purified your system with vegetables, fruits and whole grains. Now we'll add free-range, organic meats and poultry, organic dairy products and sustainably grown seafood to your diet to create maximum energy throughout the day.

The foods you consume this week will also help reset your body's sleep cycle. Remember that in chapter 6, I described how to change your environment to set the mood for better quality—and sufficient—sleep. The 21-Day Detox plan is designed to help you sleep longer, and better, than you have before. The diet additions in Phase 2 will further improve and enhance your sleep.

During this week, you'll consume about 150 more lean calories a day than in Phase 1, taking your total to about 1,600 calories a day.

Plan Ahead for Simple Meals

Just as you stocked up with grains last week, I suggest you keep some simple protein options on hand. Pick up frozen salmon, whitefish fillets and frozen shrimp, and buy a package of organic chicken breasts for fast, simple protein options. I find it helpful to make my proteins at the beginning of the week and then keep them refrigerated until I need them.

You'll note that many of these recipes call for grilled proteins; this is a quick way to prepare meat, poultry and seafood. Grill your protein in a broiler for tasty, healthful meats. To prepare ground meat, brown in a pan.

These high-protein foods include:

- Seafood (for example, salmon, tuna, shrimp, mahi mahi)
- Eggs
- Turkey
- Chicken
- Lean grass-fed beef
- Organic low-fat Greek yogurt
- Organic low-fat cottage cheese
- Organic feta cheese

You know that protein is essential to build muscle, but it also plays a vital role in helping you maintain steady energy levels and regulating optimal hormone levels. Protein also helps your body produce tryptophan, which induces sleep. I've carefully selected the foods you'll eat in this chapter for their fat-burning and balancing nature. Note that all are high in protein, which naturally

Metabolism-Boosting Spices

To help boost your metabolism, all these recipes include my top spices that will balance insulin and help burn fat. These spices include:

- Cinnamon
- Cardamom
- Cayenne
- Turmeric
- Ginger
- Mustard seed
- Black pepper
- Ginseng root
- Cumin
- Dandelion root

You'll find recommended spice suggestions in the following pages.

boosts your metabolism as your body expends more energy to digest and process protein than fats or carbohydrates. The additional protein also helps you build more lean muscle tissue, which accelerates your metabolism because muscle is more metabolically active—meaning it burns more calories all the time—than fat tissue.

Suggested Proteins

Keep in mind that these lean meat pairings are just a suggestion. If you are a fish lover, sustainable fish and seafood are the preferred protein source, so feel free to add fish to any dish instead of meat or poultry. Just make sure that your proteins have been organically grown and/or produced, and, if possible, sustainably farmed. Beef should be organic and grass-fed, if possible, for the highest nutrient quality.

THE MEAL PLAN

During the week, you'll have the same power smoothies for breakfast as last week (see pages 149–154), and choose from the same snack list (see pages 155–160). However, *you'll add clean animal protein sources to both your lunches and dinners* to provide your body with additional protein to build lean muscle and power up your metabolism.

LUNCH AND DINNER

Remember, you have 21 base lunches and 21 base dinners to choose from. Take a look at pages 164–182 to choose your favorites; just remember that variety is key for weight management and overall health. You will choose your base meal and add about three ounces (about the size of a deck of cards) of lean protein to it. I've given suggestions for each lunch and dinner, but feel free to choose other three-ounce portions of protein instead. Each recipe also includes an additional metabolism-boosting spice.

LUNCHES

1 Sun-Dried Tomato Hummus Sandwich (see recipe on page 164)
Suggested protein: 3 slices (approximately 3 ounces) turkey added to sandwich.
Spice to add: ½ teaspoon cardamom, added to hummus.

2 Orange-Strawberry Salad (see recipe on page 165)
Suggested protein: about 15 small shrimp, added to salad.
Spice to add: ½ teaspoon black pepper, added to salad dressing.

3 Chopped Italian Salad (see recipe on page 165)
Suggested protein: 3 ounces canned tuna in water, added to salad.
Spice to add: ½ teaspoon mustard seed, ground, added to salad dressing.

4 Asian Peanut Salad (see recipe on page 165)
Suggested protein: 3 ounces chicken breast, shredded, added to salad.
Spice to add: ½ teaspoon ginseng root, added to salad dressing.

5 Greek Wrap (see recipe on page 166)
Suggested protein: 3 ounces salmon, added to wrap.
Spice to add: ½ teaspoon cardamom, added to salad dressing.

6 Guacamole Wrap (see recipe on page 166)
Suggested protein: 3 ounces chicken breast, added to wrap.
Spice to add: ½ teaspoon cumin, sprinkled on pine nuts.

7 Pear and Bell Pepper Salad (see recipe on page 167)
Suggested protein: 3 ounces chicken breast, added to salad.
Spice to add: ½ teaspoon black pepper, added to salad dressing.

Fast Seafood

In some of the recipes, I've suggested grilling seafood if you choose that as a protein. Grilling is fast and easy, but other healthy preparation options include baking and sautéing. To bake fish such as salmon, mahi mahi or tuna, preheat your oven to 400°F. Place fish on a nonstick baking pan (or use no-calorie, nonstick spray) and add a dash of salt and pepper for taste. Bake for about 18 minutes, or until it flakes when you put a fork through it.

To sauté fish, place a sauté pan over high heat. Add a little olive oil to the pan, add the fish or seafood (shrimp sautés easily), and cook for about three to four minutes on each side.

8 Strawberry and Kale Salad (see recipe on page 167)
Suggested protein: about 15 small shrimp, added to salad.
Spice to add: ½ teaspoon cinnamon, sprinkled on walnuts before toasting.

9 Artichoke Salad (see recipe on page 167)
Suggested protein: 3 slices turkey (approximately 3 ounces), cut into strips, added to salad.
Spice to add: ½ teaspoon turmeric, added to salad dressing.

10 Black-Bean Tortillas with Pico de Gallo (see recipe on page 168)
Suggested protein: 3 ounces mahi mahi, added to tortillas.
Spice to add: ½ teaspoon dandelion root powder, added to Pico de Gallo.

11 Avocado Sandwich (see recipe on page 168)
Suggested protein: 3 ounces grilled chicken breast, shredded, added to sandwich.
Spice to add: ½ teaspoon cumin, mixed in with avocado and chicken.

12 Simple Greek Salad (see recipe on page 168)
Suggested protein: 3 ounces canned tuna in water, added to salad.
Spice to add: ½ teaspoon turmeric, added to salad dressing.

13 Tex-Mex Salad (see recipe on page 169)
Suggested protein: 3 ounces chicken breast, shredded or chopped, added to salad.
Spice to add: ½ teaspoon cumin, added to salad dressing.

14 Thai Lettuce Wrap (see recipe on page 169)
Suggested protein: about 15 small shrimp, added to wrap.
Spice to add: ¼ teaspoon ginseng root, added to salad dressing.

15 Smashed White Bean and Avocado Sandwich (see recipe on page 169)
Suggested protein: 3 turkey slices or 3 ounces turkey, added to sandwich.
Spice to add: ¼ teaspoon cardamom, added to white bean mash.

16 Lettuce and Tomato Sandwich on a Bagel (see recipe on page 170)
Suggested protein: 3 ounces tuna, added to sandwich.
Spice to add: ¼ teaspoon cayenne, added to tuna.

17 Potato Wrap (see recipe on page 170)
Suggested protein: 3 ounces chicken breast, added to wrap.
Spice to add: ½ teaspoon mustard seed, ground, sprinkled over chicken.

18 Cold Quinoa Salad (see recipe on page 171)
Suggested protein: about 15 shrimp, added to salad.
Spice to add: ½ teaspoon cinnamon, rubbed onto shrimp before cooking.

19 Asian-Inspired Salad (see recipe on page 171)
Suggested protein: 3 ounces salmon, added to salad.
Spice to add: ¼ teaspoon ginseng root, added to salad dressing.

20 Tex-Mex Wrap (see recipe on page 171)
Suggested protein: 3 ounces chicken breast, added to wrap.
Spice to add: ½ teaspoon cumin, added to black beans, corn and rice.

21 Brown Rice and Chickpea Salad (see recipe on page 171)
Suggested protein: 3 ounces chicken breast, added to salad.
Spice to add: ½ teaspoon turmeric, added to dressing.

DINNERS

The dinner recipes are taken from your base diet on pages 172–182. Once again, I've suggested proteins for each recipe, and added thermogenic spices to some recipes to boost your body's fat-burning potential.

Note that each of these recipes is made to serve four people. Simply add one serving of protein per individual for each meal, as suggested below.

1 Potato and Veggie Skillet (see recipe on page 172)
Suggested protein: 4 three-ounce pieces salmon.
Spice to add: ½ teaspoon cardamom, added to potatoes and vegetables.

2 Broccoli and Wild Rice (see recipe on page 173)
Suggested protein: 4 three-ounce pieces chicken breast.
Spice to add: ½ teaspoon black pepper, added to broccoli, rice and onion mixture.

3 Sweet Pea Pasta with Olive Oil (see recipe on page 173)
Suggested protein: 4 cups shrimp.
Spice to add: 1 teaspoon turmeric, added to olive oil.

4 Turkey Burger and Grilled Asparagus (see recipe for Portabella Burger on page 174)
Suggested protein: substitute 1 pound extra-lean ground turkey breast for portabella mushrooms. Shape into four patties, add salt and pepper and grill until cooked through.

5 Indonesian Peanut Rice (see recipe on page 174)
Suggested protein: 4 cups shrimp.
Spice to add: ¼ teaspoon ginseng root, added to sauce.

6 Cuban-Style Rice and Beans with Mango (see recipe on page 175)
Suggested protein: 4 three-ounce pieces chicken breast, grilled.
Spice to add: 1 teaspoon paprika, rubbed on chicken before grilling.

7 Spinach and Bean Casserole (see recipe on page 175)
Suggested protein: 4 three-ounce pieces mahi mahi, grilled or baked.
Spice to add: ½ teaspoon mustard seed, ground, added to casserole.

8 Brussels Sprouts Ragout (see recipe on page 176)
Suggested protein: 4 three-ounce pieces mahi mahi.
Spice to add: ¼ teaspoon cayenne, added to ragout.

9 Quinoa with Sun-Dried Tomatoes (see recipe on page 176)
Suggested protein: 4 three-ounce pieces halibut.
Spice to add: ¼ teaspoon cardamom, added to quinoa.

10 Wild Rice Skillet (see recipe on page 177)
Suggested protein: 4 three-ounce pieces chicken breast.
Spice to add: ½ teaspoon black pepper, added to rice.

11 Pasta Primavera (see recipe on page 177)
Suggested protein: 4 cups shrimp.
Spice to add: 1 teaspoon turmeric, added to pasta with salt, pepper and basil.

12 Beef Fajitas (see recipe for Veggie Fajitas on page 178)
Suggested protein: 12 ounces lean beef, grilled, sliced and added to fajitas.
Spice to add: 1 teaspoon black pepper, added to vegetables.

13 Penne with Tomatoes and Kale (see recipe on page 178)
Suggested protein: 4 three-ounce pieces grilled tilapia.
Spice to add: 1 teaspoon cumin, rubbed onto tilapia before grilling.

14 Turkey Chili (see recipe for Vegan Chili on page 179)
Suggested protein: 12 ounces lean ground turkey, browned.
Spice to add: 2 teaspoons cumin, added to chili.

15 Black Bean-Topped Sweet Potatoes (see recipe on page 179)
Suggested protein: 12 ounces lean beef.
Spice to add: 1 teaspoon cayenne, added to black bean stuffing.

16 Spinach and Artichoke Pasta Bake (see recipe on page 180)
Suggested protein: 4 three-ounce pieces salmon.
Spice to add: ½ teaspoon cumin, added to vegetables before baking.

17 Pepper and Cauliflower Hash (see recipe on page 180)
Suggested protein: 4 eggs. Whisk well and add to vegetables after cooking. Bake for 10 minutes at 350°F until eggs are cooked through. Season with salt and pepper. Add basil and pine nuts and serve.
Spice to add: ½ teaspoon mustard seed, ground, added to peppers.

18 Cream of Broccoli and Pistachio Soup (see recipe on page 181)
Suggested protein: 4 three-ounce pieces sea bass.
Spice to add: ¼ teaspoon cardamom, added to soup.

19 Stuffed Peppers (see recipe on page 181)
Suggested protein: 4 three-ounce pieces salmon.
Spice to add: 1 teaspoon turmeric, added to pepper stuffing.

20 Veggie Couscous with Chicken (see recipe for Veggie Couscous on page 182)
Suggested protein: 4 three-ounce pieces chicken breast.
Spice to add: 1 teaspoon cumin, added to couscous.

21 Simple Chicken Soup (see recipe for Veggie Soup on page 182)
Suggested protein: 12 ounces chicken breast, grilled or roasted. Cut into cubes before adding to soup.
Spice to add: 2 teaspoons cayenne, added to soup.

MENU PLAN

Here's what a week of meals might look like for Phase 2:

MONDAY (DAY 1)

Breakfast: Berry Smoothie (see recipe on page 149)

Snack: Baba Ghanoush and Cucumber (see recipe on page 156)

Lunch: Thai Lettuce Wrap (see recipe on page 218)

Snack: Baked Chips with Pico de Gallo (see recipe on page 157)

Dinner: Pepper and Cauliflower Hash (see recipe on page 221)

After Dinner: Ginger Detox Tea (see recipe on page 147)

TUESDAY (DAY 2)

Breakfast: Avocado-Pear Smoothie (see recipe on page 151)

Snack: Almond Butter and Coconut Apple (see recipe on page 160)

Lunch: Greek Wrap (see recipe on page 217)

Snack: Nutty Melon (see recipe on page 155)

Dinner: Potato and Veggie Skillet (see recipe on page 219)

After Dinner: Ginger Detox Tea (see recipe on page 147)

WEDNESDAY (DAY 3)

Breakfast: Apple Smoothie (see recipe on page 151)

Snack: Peach Bread (see recipe on page 159)

Lunch: Artichoke Salad (see recipe on page 218)

Snack: Guacamole and Chips (see recipe on page 160)

Dinner: Beef Fajitas (see recipe on page 220)

After Dinner: Ginger Detox Tea (see recipe on page 147)

THURSDAY (DAY 4)

Breakfast:	Melon Smoothie (see recipe on page 150)
Snack:	Peanut Butter and Banana Rice Cake (see recipe on page 156)
Lunch:	Black Bean Tortillas with Pico de Gallo (see recipe on page 218)
Snack:	Frozen Grapes with Pumpkin Seeds (see recipe on page 159)
Dinner:	Sweet Pea Pasta with Shrimp and Olive Oil (see recipe on page 219)
After Dinner:	Ginger Detox Tea (see recipe on page 147)

FRIDAY (DAY 5)

Breakfast:	Beet Smoothie (see recipe on page 149)
Snack:	Almond Butter and Celery (see recipe on page 156)
Lunch:	Avocado Sandwich (see recipe on page 218)
Snack:	Spicy Toasted Chickpeas (see recipe on page 157)
Dinner:	Turkey Burger with Grilled Asparagus (see recipe on page 220)
After Dinner:	Ginger Detox Tea (see recipe on page 147)

SATURDAY (DAY 6)

Breakfast:	Citrus Smoothie (see recipe on page 149)
Snack:	Tomato with Pine Nuts (see recipe on page 156)
Lunch:	Asian Peanut Salad (see recipe on page 217)
Snack:	Honey Pear (see recipe on page 158)
Dinner:	Broccoli and Wild Rice (see recipe on page 219)
After Dinner:	Ginger Detox Tea (see recipe on page 147)

SUNDAY (DAY 7)

Breakfast:	Strawberries and Chocolate Smoothie (see recipe on page 150)
Snack:	Carrots/Celery and Hummus (see recipe on page 155)
Lunch:	Guacamole Wrap (see recipe on page 217)
Snack:	Cinnamon-Apple Slices (see recipe on page 159)
Dinner:	Turkey Chili (see recipe on page 221)
After Dinner:	Ginger Detox Tea (see recipe on page 147)

EXERCISE: BURN ROUTINE

Last week, your workouts were relatively simple—you performed four sets of four different exercises for two different body parts. Those basic movements will be incorporated in this week's workout. The main difference is that you will be performing multijoint or compound moves. You will be working your upper body and lower body simultaneously. Besides really making you lean, engagement of more muscles means you are automatically burning extra calories with every move.

These compound moves drive your body into the cardio zone, giving you both strength training and cardio at once, and turning you into a fat-burning machine. It's like two workouts in one. This style of anabolic aerobics will burn the most fat calories while strengthening muscle cells. These workouts will ignite the maximum amount of muscle fibers at once, incinerating fat, sending energy through the roof and deepening sleep.

Multijoint movements force the heart to pump to upper and lower extremities, keeping you in a heightened cardiovascular zone. No other exercise style has the fat-burning potential of multijoint movements.

Extra Training Benefits

Research shows that this style of training doesn't just burn calories during workouts, it also carries over to promote continuous fat-burning for 8 to 12 hours postworkout.

This week you'll perform two sets of four exercises (10 repetitions each) back to back, with no rest. Because you're moving multiple joints at the same time, you will use your core and your balance more than you did in the previous two phases. This will improve joint stability and core strength.

Phase 2 Workout: BURN

MONDAY/THURSDAY

Squat/Biceps Curl: 10 reps/2 sets

Bridge/Flat Press: 10 reps/2 sets

Plié Squat with Hammer Curl: 10 reps/2 sets

Bridge/Flat Dumbbell Fly: 10 reps/2 sets

TUESDAY/FRIDAY

Deadlift with Bent-Over Row: 10 reps/2 sets

Lunge with Kickback: 10 reps/2 sets

Alternating Lunge with Reverse Grip Row: 10 reps/2 sets

Backward Lunge with Standing Head-Banger: 10 reps/2 sets

WEDNESDAY/SATURDAY

Side Lunge with Lateral Raise: 10 reps/2 sets

Close Squat/Hammer: 10 reps/2 sets

Squat with WV: 10 reps/2 sets

Plié Squat with Military Press: 10 reps/2 sets

SUNDAY

Rest Day

HERE'S THE WORKOUT
MONDAY/THURSDAY

SQUAT/BICEPS CURL

Stand with your feet under your hips, toes pointed slightly out, dumbbells in front, knuckles facing backward. Engage your abdominal muscles and bend your knees to push your bottom back and down. As you squat, bend your arms to curl the dumbbells toward your shoulders. Then return your hands to your sides as you rise.

10REPS
X 2SETS

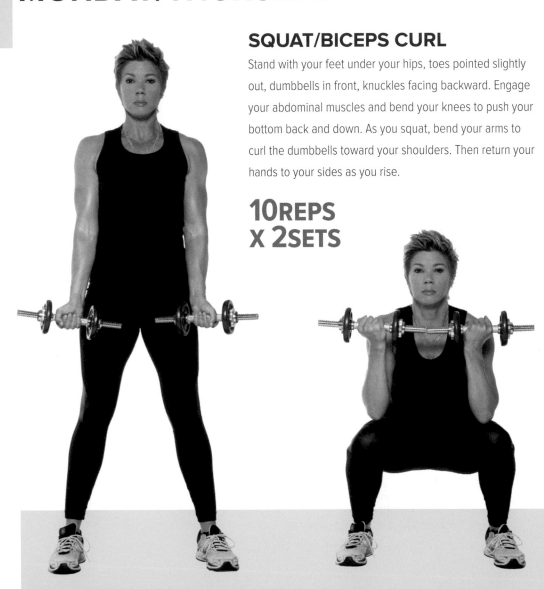

BRIDGE/FLAT PRESS

Lie on your back on the floor, dumbbells in both hands with your knuckles facing the ceiling, elbows making a 90-degree angle. Your feet should be under your knees and your abs braced. Engage your chest muscles and press the weights toward the ceiling, while lifting your pelvis to make a bridge. Lower your pelvis and arms to the starting position. That's one rep.

10REPS X 2SETS

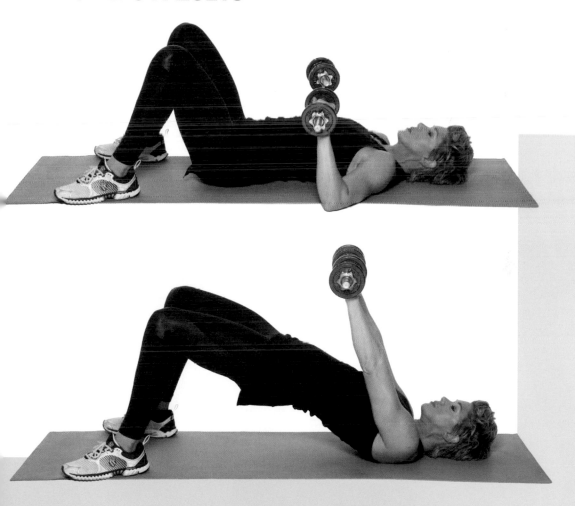

MONDAY/THURSDAY
CONTINUED

PLIÉ SQUAT WITH HAMMER CURL

Stand with your feet about 12 inches outside your hips, toes pointed slightly out, holding dumbbells in both hands with your knuckles facing out. Engage your abdominal muscles (imagine pulling them back toward your spine) and, keeping your chest up, bend your knees to push your bottom back and down. At the same time, bend your arms to bring the dumbbells toward your shoulders, keeping your knuckles facing out. Return to the starting position, lowering the dumbbells as you rise.

10REPS X 2SETS

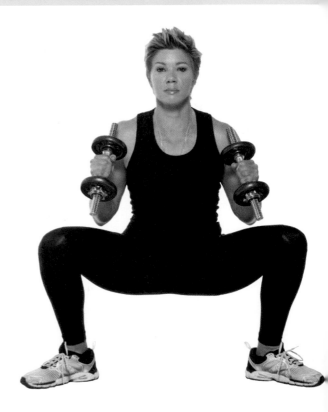

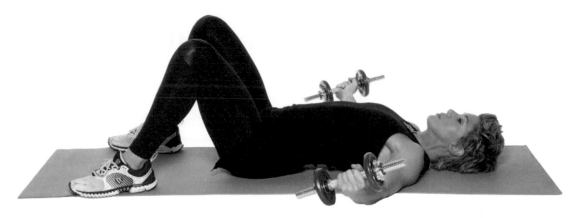

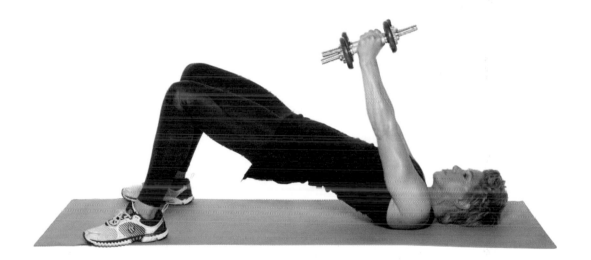

BRIDGE/FLAT DUMBBELL FLY

Lie on your back on a weight bench or on the floor, dumbbells in both hands with your arms open. Your feet should be hip-width apart, knees bent and your abs braced. Lift your hips so your torso forms a straight line (and creates a bridge) as you close your arms and raise them above your chest. Lower your hips and your arms to the starting postion.

10 REPS X 2 SETS

TUESDAY/FRIDAY

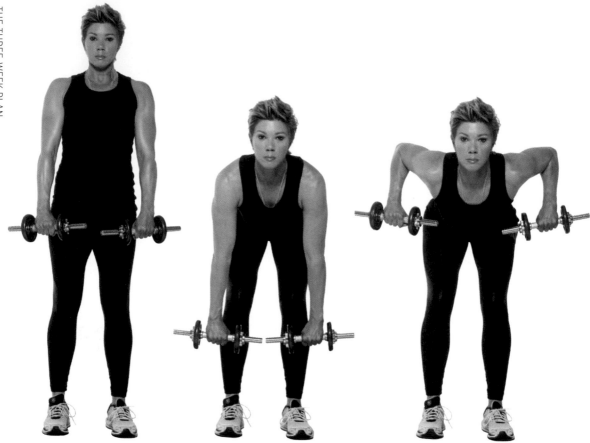

DEADLIFT WITH BENT-OVER ROW

Hold dumbbells in front of your thighs, knuckles facing forward, feet under your hips. Hinge forward until your back is nearly parallel to the ground, bending your knees slightly, and then pull the dumbbells up toward your navel. Slowly lower the weights back down and then rise for the next rep.

10REPS X 2SETS

BACKWARD LUNGE WITH KICKBACK

Stand with your feet directly under your hips, dumbbells in hands. Step backward with your right leg so that your knee is about 5 inches from the ground. As you step backward, straighten your arms to your sides. Perform each lunge and kickback simultaneously on each side, then switch sides. That's one rep.

20REPS
X 2SETS

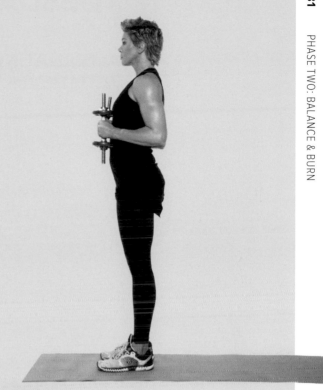

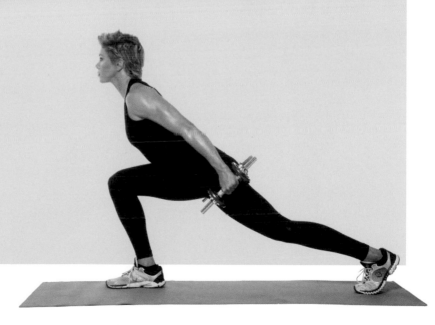

TUESDAY/FRIDAY

CONTINUED

ALTERNATING LUNGE
WITH REVERSE GRIP ROW

Hold dumbbells in front of your thighs, knuckles facing your body, feet under your hips, toes pointed slightly out. Step forward with your right leg. As you lower your left knee toward the ground, pull your arms up toward your body. Alternate stepping forward with your left leg and lowering your right knee toward the ground as you row your arms up toward your body. That's one rep.

10REPS x 2SETS

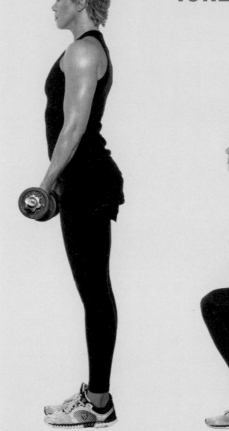
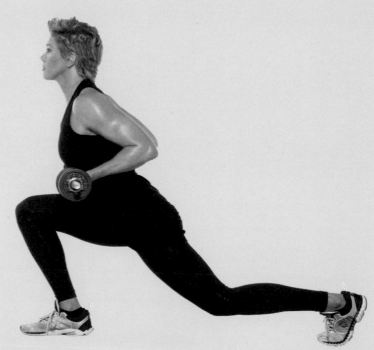

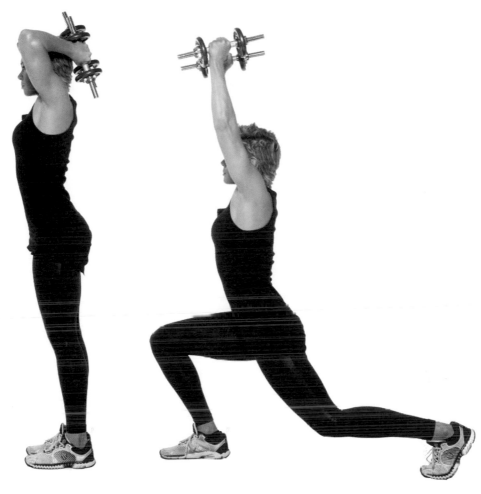

BACKWARD LUNGE WITH STANDING HEAD-BANGER

Stand with your feet directly under your hips, holding dumbbells behind your head. Step forward with your right leg. As you lower your left knee toward the ground, straighten dumbbells above your head. Slowly extend your arms back to the original position as you bring your left knee back to the original position. Repeat, stepping forward with your left leg and lowering your right knee to the ground as you complete another head-banger. That's one rep.

10REPS X 2SETS

WEDNESDAY/SATURDAY

SIDE LUNGE WITH LATERAL RAISE

Stand with your feet together, holding dumbbells in both hands with your elbows straight. Engage your abdominal muscles (imagine pulling them back toward your spine) and, keeping your chest up, lunge to the side. At the same time, lift your arms at your sides to shoulder height. Lower your arms as you return to the starting position, then repeat on the opposite side. That's one rep.

10REPS X 2SETS

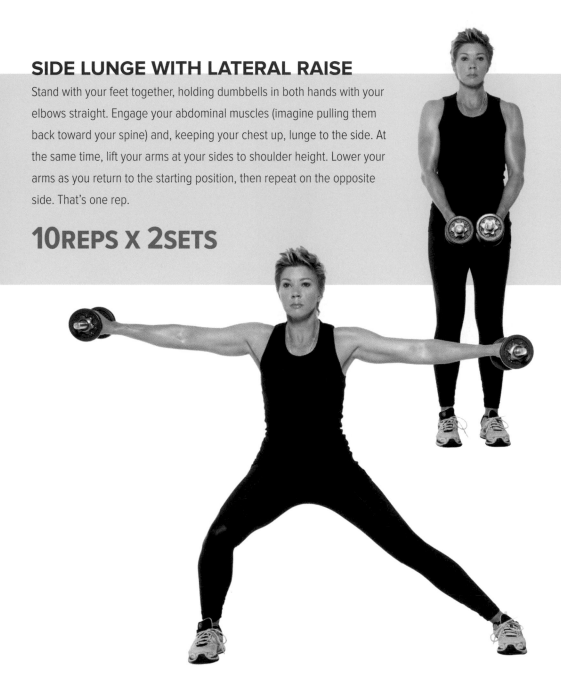

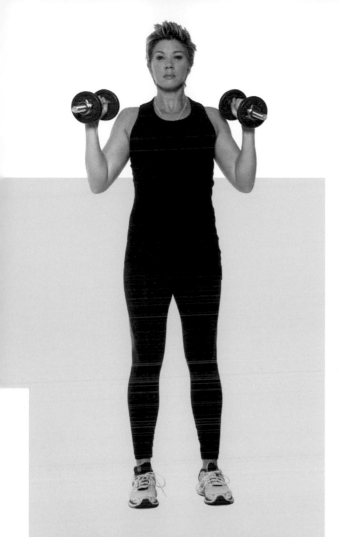

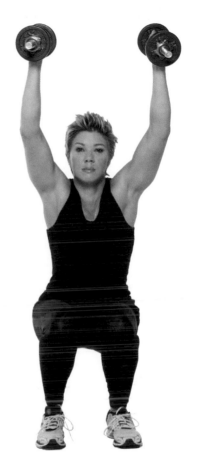

CLOSE SQUAT/HAMMER

Stand with your feet directly under your hips, dumbbells in your hands at shoulder height. Engage your abdominal muscles (imagine pulling them back toward your spine) and, keeping your chest up, lower yourself into a squatting position while moving the dumbbells directly above your head.

10REPS X 2SETS

WEDNESDAY/SATURDAY
CONTINUED

SQUAT WITH WV

Stand with your feet just outside your hips, toes pointed slightly out, dumbbells in both hands, arms bent and at your sides, knuckles facing out. (Your arms will form the letter *W*.) Engage your abdominal muscles (imagine pulling them back toward your spine) and, keeping your chest up, bend your knees to push your bottom back and down. As you squat, simultaneously press the dumbbells up and out in a slight diagonal so that your arms are straight, and they now make the letter *V*. Straighten your legs and bring your arms back to the original *W* position at the same time.

10REPS x 2SETS

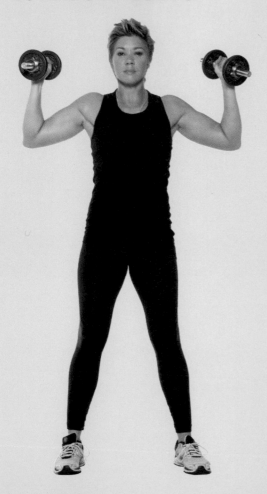

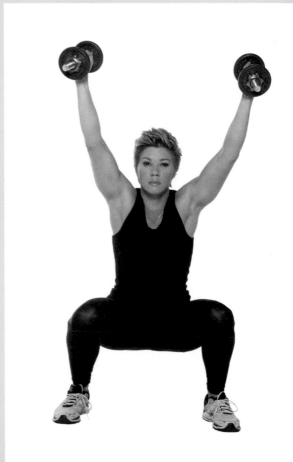

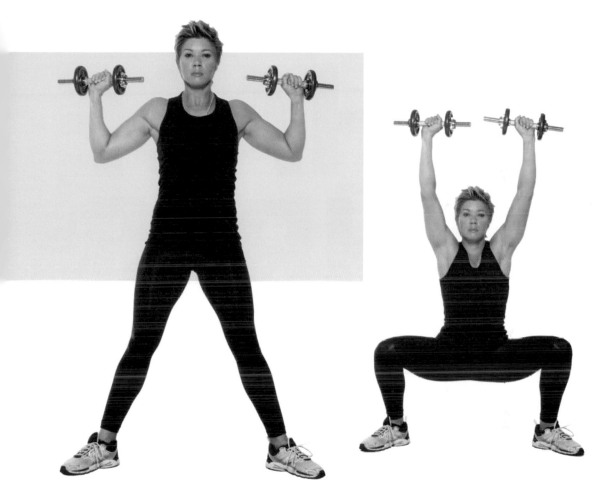

PLIÉ SQUAT WITH MILITARY PRESS

Stand with your feet wide apart, toes pointed out, holding dumbbells at shoulder height, knuckles facing your shoulders. Engage your abdominal muscles and bend your knees to push your bottom back and down. Your knees will track over your second and third toes while staying behind your toes. As you squat, press the dumbbells up slightly in front of your shoulders. Lower your arms as you straighten your legs to return to the starting position.

10REPS X 2SETS

CHAPTER NINE

PHASE THREE: LEAN & MEAN

Welcome to my personal eating and training program! Over the next 7 days, you will eat and train exactly the way I do. After the past 14 days, your internal chemistry has completely changed. You are clean and energetic. You should be feeling pretty good about yourself!

The cells and tissues of the body have been primed, cleansed and balanced, and are ready for the ultimate in muscle shaping and strengthening. Metabolic and mood hormones have been recalibrated and you've retuned your body clock; you feel calmer, you're sleeping better and your motivation is off the chart. It's time to take it up a notch and engineer your peak form, not just for the following week, but for life. Some diets give you a "maintenance" plan to follow—but this is a lifestyle that will give you good health and energy for life!

THE LEAN PLAN (MEAL TIMING)

We have a saying in the bodybuilding community: "The body is made in the kitchen." Every trainer knows that nutrition and the timing of meals is absolutely key to having a toned, beautiful body. Under the Lean Plan, you will continue eating portions of meals similar to those in the previous chapter. The difference is that now you will eat meals or snacks within 30 minutes of your workouts and you will eat a snack or meal containing protein, fat and carbs within 30 minutes postworkout. The snack should contain proteins, fat and fruit carbs. Your calories are about 1,800 per day, and the amount of meals and snacks remain the same—five each day. But instead of eating every two to three hours, you will be timing meals and snacks around training.

Here are suggested eating times for Phase 3, assuming that you train in the morning. If you don't, remember to eat a meal and snack within 30 minutes pre-train and post-train.

8:00 a.m.	Breakfast
8:30 a.m.	Train
9:30 a.m.	Postworkout Snack
11:30 a.m.	Snack
1:00 p.m.	Lunch
3:00 – 4:00 p.m.	Snack
6:00 p.m.	Dinner

If you are trying to lose weight, you will, because of the highly thermogenic properties of the foods selected. Every time you eat, your body's metabolism rises as you digest the food you've consumed, and this creates heat, called thermogenesis. Some foods require more energy to digest, which means they generate more heat and are more metabolically active than others. Fat and carbs are more readily broken down by your body than protein, which requires more energy to digest and use.

Protein is the building block of muscle, which is what keeps you lean, strong and sexy. When we eat to optimize muscle tissue, we accelerate metabolism and fat-burning, which literally works to lean out the body. Proteins are also incredibly thermogenic, meaning they shift your metabolic furnace into maximum burning mode. As you did in Phase 1 and Phase 2, you'll also continue to consume proteins, fruits, whole grains, veggies and fats. These, together with healthy fats and clean proteins, will boost daytime power and keep energy levels steady and strong.

Adding More Protein

In Phase 3, you will add a scoop of whey isolate protein to your power smoothie. Choose the all-natural kind. Look for no hormones or artificial ingredients on the label and make sure it has at least 25 grams of protein per serving.

Timing Your Postworkout Snack

If you train in the morning, your power smoothie with whey protein meets the requirements for muscle growth. Simply follow that exercise with a postworkout snack. If you train after work, make sure you have your portable snack preworkout. Then just eat your dinner after your workout.

Your snacks are timed around your workouts and will feed hungry muscles that need this fuel for toning. On days when you don't work out, you will eat the way you did in Phase 1 and Phase 2. If you choose not to work out with this program, then stick to the Balance and Burn meals.

POSTWORKOUT SNACKS

For your postworkout snack, you'll want to consume a snack that contains protein, carbs and a little healthy fat. Here are some suggestions:

+ 1 cup cantaloupe with 1 cup Greek low-fat yogurt and 10 pistachios

+ 3 slices turkey with a banana and 5 macadamia nuts

+ 1 hard-boiled egg with a medium pear and 5 walnuts

+ 1 cup pineapple chunks with 1 tablespoon pine nuts and 3 slices of beef

+ 3 slices chicken breast or ham on a slice of whole-grain bread with a small peach

+ 1 tablespoon almond butter on an apple with a hard-boiled egg

+ 1 cup low-fat cottage cheese with a tangerine and 10 almonds

As you did with the meals, experiment to find your favorite postworkout snack. I care less about which protein/fruit combo you choose and more about the timing of this postworkout mini-meal.

MENU PLAN

Here is a sample week based on a morning workout routine:

MONDAY (DAY 1)

Breakfast:	Blueberry-Banana Smoothie (see recipe on page 150)
Postworkout Snack:	1 cup cantaloupe with 1 cup Greek low-fat yogurt and 10 pistachios
Snack:	Baba Ghanoush and Cucumber (see recipe on page 156)
Lunch:	Strawberry and Kale Salad (see recipe on page 218)
Snack:	Nutty Melon (see recipe on page 155)
Dinner:	Spinach and Artichoke Pasta Bake (see recipe on page 221)
After Dinner:	Ginger Detox Tea (see recipe on page 147)

TUESDAY (DAY 2)

Breakfast:	Apple Pie Smoothie (see recipe on page 153)
Postworkout Snack:	3 slices turkey with a banana and 5 macadamia nuts
Snack:	Bell Peppers with Sweet Potato Hummus (see recipe on page 158)
Lunch:	Smashed White Bean and Avocado Sandwich (see recipe on page 218)
Snack:	Almond Butter and Coconut Apple (see recipe on page 160)
Dinner:	Brussels Sprouts Ragout (see recipe on page 220)
After Dinner:	Ginger Detox Tea (see recipe on page 147)

WEDNESDAY (DAY 3)

Breakfast: Pineapple Smoothie (see recipe on page 149)

Postworkout Snack: 1 hard-boiled egg with a medium pear and 5 walnuts

Snack: Spicy Avocado (see recipe on page 159)

Lunch: Sun-Dried Tomato Hummus Sandwich (see recipe on page 217)

Snack: Baked Chips with Pico de Gallo (see recipe on page 157)

Dinner: Wild Rice Skillet (see recipe on page 220)

After Dinner: Ginger Detox Tea (see recipe on page 147)

THURSDAY (DAY 4)

Breakfast: Orange Smoothie (see recipe on page 150)

Postworkout Snack: 1 cup pineapple chunks with 1 tablespoon pine nuts and 3 slices lean beef

Snack: Artichoke Dip (see recipe on page 160)

Lunch: Potato Wrap (see recipe on page 218)

Snack: Peanut Butter and Banana Rice Cake (see recipe on page 156)

Dinner: Cream of Broccoli and Pistachio Soup (see recipe on page 221)

After Dinner: Ginger Detox Tea (see recipe on page 147)

FRIDAY (DAY 5)

Breakfast: Banana-Avocado Smoothie (see recipe on page 152)

Postworkout Snack: 3 slices chicken breast or ham on a slice of whole-grain bread with a small peach

Snack: Almond-Kale Chips (see recipe on page 158)

Lunch: Asian Peanut Salad (see recipe on page 217)

Snack: Quick Wrap (see recipe on page 159)

Dinner: Stuffed Peppers (see recipe on page 221)

After Dinner: Ginger Detox Tea (see recipe on page 147)

SATURDAY (DAY 6)

Breakfast:	Cherry-Grapefruit Smoothie (see recipe on page 153)
Postworkout Snack:	1 tablespoon almond butter on an apple with a hard-boiled egg
Snack:	Peach Bread (see recipe on page 159)
Lunch:	Tex-Mex Salad (see recipe on page 218)
Snack:	Carrots/Celery and Hummus and Honey Pear (see recipes on page 155 and 158)
Dinner:	Simple Chicken Soup (see recipe on page 221)
After Dinner:	Ginger Detox Tea (see recipe on page 147)

SUNDAY (DAY 7)

Breakfast:	Aloha Smoothie (see recipe on page 153)
Postworkout Snack:	1 cup low-fat cottage cheese with a tangerine and 10 almonds
Snack:	Spicy Toasted Chickpeas (see recipe on page 157)
Lunch:	Orange-Strawberry Salad and Guacamole Wrap (see recipes on page 217)
Snack:	Cinnamon-Apple Slices (see recipe on page 159)
Dinner:	Turkey Chili (see recipe on page 221)
After Dinner:	Ginger Detox Tea (see recipe on page 147)

The diet you've been following has been strategically customized to meet the demands of your recharged body from now until forever! Each meal has been designed to cause a different chemical reaction at different times of the day. For example, the breakfasts and lunches you've been consuming contain energy-sustaining foods, while dinners contain foods that naturally trigger dopamine and serotonin, the body's natural relaxant.

EXERCISE: MEAN ROUTINE

During Phase 1, you used supersets and slow, controlled form to start priming your muscles for the coming workouts. During Phase 2, you performed compound movements to accelerate caloric burn and boost your metabolism, along with building muscle. Now, in Phase 3, you'll use Power Ladders, my favorite and most body-transforming training method. You've done almost all these moves already, and any new ones have descriptions.

Power Ladders are the ultimate workout for power, strength and endurance. During these next seven days (and from now on), you'll become an athlete, igniting a fire during your workouts that will carry through to your everyday life. Now you're ready to complete very specific functional exercises with perfect form to complete fatigue in order to yield the highest efficiency in everyday life.

Each workout provides a powerful dose of youth hormones, which will build muscle, produce the highest-quality sleep and energy, and bring more oxygen to the skin, giving you a bright, energized and attractive appearance. Mood-enhancing hormones are tripled, giving you a feeling of confidence and well-being. And sleep hormones will be produced in abundance, allowing for a more restful sleep.

So how do you perform a ladder? It's simple. You start with 1 repetition of each exercise done back to back with no rest and then climb up the ladder until you reach 10 reps. So for example: 1 push-up/1 hammer curl; 2 push-ups/ 2 hammer curls, 3 push-ups/3 hammer curls and so on until you reach 10. You're going to aim for a total of 55 reps of each exercise, after climbing down the ladder, so get ready to be challenged! These exercises are tough, so rest 1–3 minutes between sets.

Phase 3 Workout: MEAN

MONDAY/THURSDAY

Push-up/Hammer Curl: 1 set, 110 total reps

Flat Dumbbell Press/Wide Curl: 1 set, 110 total reps

Flat Dumbbell Fly/Close Curl : 1 set, 110 total reps

TUESDAY/FRIDAY

Bent Row/Lying Down Head-Banger: 1 set, 110 total reps

Wide Row/Kickback: 1 set, 110 total reps

Alternating Row/Standing Head-Banger: 1 set, 110 total reps

WEDNESDAY/SATURDAY

Squat/Lateral Raise: 1 set, 110 total reps

Plié Squat/Arnold Press: 1 set, 110 total reps

Front Lunge/WV: 1 set, 110 total reps

SUNDAY

Rest Day

HERE'S THE WORKOUT

MONDAY/THURSDAY

Today's workout moves focus on the chest and biceps. All moves should look familiar, except for the push-up. You may already know how to perform this move. If not, follow this simple step:

Lie facedown, with your hands under your shoulders, and your weight on your knees (called a modified push-up) or on your toes. Push yourself up, keeping your abs engaged and your body in a straight line, and then lower yourself until your elbows make a 90-degree angle. Push back up. That's one rep.

So here is today's ladder workout:

MON/THUR

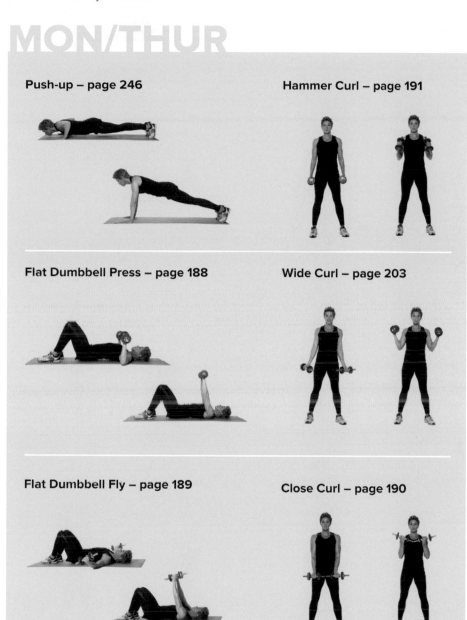

Push-up – page 246

Hammer Curl – page 191

Flat Dumbbell Press – page 188

Wide Curl – page 203

Flat Dumbbell Fly – page 189

Close Curl – page 190

TUESDAY/FRIDAY

Today's workout focuses on the back and triceps.

You'll do a ladder of the following:

TUES/FRI

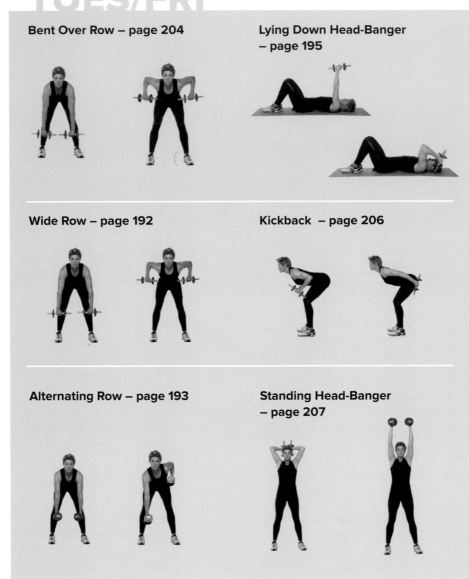

Bent Over Row – page 204

Lying Down Head-Banger – page 195

Wide Row – page 192

Kickback – page 206

Alternating Row – page 193

Standing Head-Banger – page 207

WEDNESDAY/SATURDAY

Today's workout focuses on the legs and shoulders.

You'll do ladders of the following:

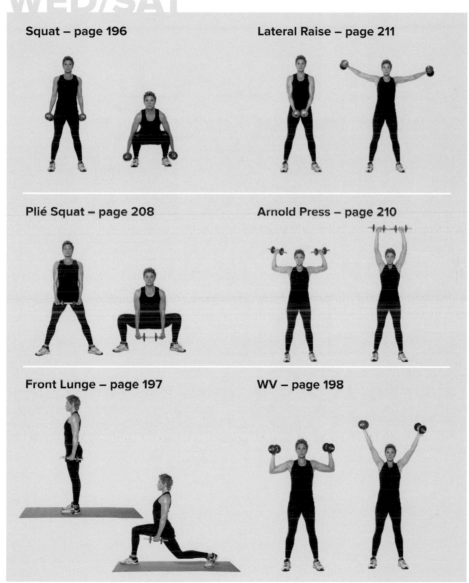

Squat – page 196

Lateral Raise – page 211

Plié Squat – page 208

Arnold Press – page 210

Front Lunge – page 197

WV – page 198

SUNDAY (REST DAY)

CHAPTER TEN

WHAT'S NEXT?

HARNESSING YOUR ENERGY TO PURSUE YOUR DREAMS

So what's next? The answer is up to you.

You now have the plan to follow for the rest of your life. You've learned how to eat to fuel your body and eliminate toxins, and how to efficiently exercise in a way that will change your body from the inside out! On days when you're not working out, follow the Balance and Burn meal plan in chapter 8. On days when you do work out, add a postworkout snack within 30 to 45 minutes of working out. As you follow the program, you'll see that your strength increases—an additional external validation of what's happening on the inside of your body!

After you've completed all three phases, you have the diet you should follow for life—and the energy to live the life you've dreamed of. It really is that simple. You should feel like a whole new you.

It's been 21 days, and in that short time, you've detoxed and rebuilt your body from the inside out. Your cells are healthy—possibly the healthiest they've been since you were a child—and your body's adrenal and thyroid function have been optimized. You're getting quality, solid sleep, and can already see a difference in the mirror. You look younger, feel clearer and your energy is powerful!

If that was all you'd gain from doing this program, that would be enough, wouldn't it? But that's literally only the beginning. You've gone from so-so to superstar, and now it's time to harness your newfound and well-deserved energy. My plan isn't meant to be an end, but a beginning.

Now you know how to eat to feed your body's cells and rebalance your internal systems. You know how to exercise to build lean muscle and fire your

My Personal Journey

When I was 18, I came to Los Angeles for school. I knew I wanted to do something great in life—I just didn't know what. At age 20, I started working out and eating healthier, and that sparked a tremendous change in me. My mind became clear. I didn't go home and watch TV all night; I wrote and painted because I had energy. These creative outlets gave me tremendous self-esteem.

My strong body gave me confidence and I carried myself like a totally different person than I had in high school. My extreme shyness dissipated and I felt socially comfortable and confident. I knew that I owed this to my healthy lifestyle. Without it, I could never have started a small business that made me a millionaire by 21. To say that fitness changed my life is an understatement. No matter what is going on in the world, I still have my health and my strong body. No breakups or financial losses can take that away from me and I am very comforted by that.

metabolism. You're getting the quality sleep you need for emotional and physical health. So what comes next? How about using that energy to pursue the dreams you've set aside, or maybe given up on, until now.

Never think of this program as depriving yourself. Think of it as giving yourself the most loving gift of all. You are ready to make better choices for yourself and, when you do, I promise the Universe will reward you.

What's Next for *You*?

Now that you know what I've been able to do, consider your own life and goals. Take some time to think about what you really want or what you're passionate about. Record your thoughts here.

1 As a child, I dreamed of:

_____

_____

_____

What do I have to do to make this a reality?

_____

_____

2 When I do this _____, I feel good about myself.

This is often a creative pursuit, such as painting or writing. Remember, you do not need training for either—it comes from the heart and practice makes perfect. So just get started!

3 If I could pursue any career, it would be to:

_____

_____

Talk about it! You will get that dream job by referral or writing a specialized, strong résumé. Remember, getting a job is a numbers game. Send your résumé out to several companies until one sticks.

4 My personal "bucket list" includes the following things:

_____

_____

Make a list and post it somewhere important. Try to cross at least one thing off your list each year.

5 I've always wanted to, but have been afraid to, try the following:

_____

_____

Not facing fear actually causes depression. As humans we are built for bravery. Ask yourself, "What is the best that can happen and what is the worst that can happen?" The "best" usually wins.

6 I'm really good at _____.
How can I start a business that uses those talents?

_____

_____

This is a great example of using your energy and passion. Whenever I start a business, this is exactly what I do!

I wrote this book because I wanted to help more people transform their lives the way I've helped thousands of others already. I know that there is nothing more satisfying and fulfilling than accomplishing a dream. You have the energy, the vitality and the good health to pursue yours, so it's now up to you!

Your body looks and feels amazing from the inside out. With your newfound energy, health and vitality, you're now able to live with intention, with purpose and with passion. That is how I live my life, and that is what I wish for you, my readers.

BIBLIOGRAPHY

CHAPTER 1

Abumrad, N., D. Piomelli, K. Yurko-Mauro, et al. "Moving Beyond 'Good Fat, Bad Fat': The Complex Roles of Dietary Lipids in Cellular Function and Health." *Advances in Nutrition* 3, no. 1 (January 2012): 60–68.

American Cancer Society. "Lifetime Risk of Developing or Dying From Cancer." http://www.cancer.org/cancer/cancerbasics/lifetime-probability-of-developing-or-dying-from-cancer (accessed November 2, 2014).

Ames, B., H. Atamna, and D. Killilea. "Mineral and Vitamin Deficiencies Can Accelerate the Mitochondrial Decay of Aging." *Science Direct. Molecular Aspects of Medicine* 26 (2005): 363–78.

Arola-Arnal, A., and C. Blade. "Proanthocynadnidins Modulate microRNA Expression in Human HepG2 cells." *PloS One* 6, no. 10 (2011): e25982.

Aseervathem, G. S., T. Sivasudha, R. Jeyadevi, and D. Arul Ananth. "Environmental Factors and Unhealthy Lifestyle Influence Oxidative Stress in Humans—An Overview." *Environmental Science and Pollution Research International* 20, no. 7 (July 2013): 4356 69.

Bendetti, D., E. Nunes, M. Sarmento, et al. "Genetic Damage in Soybean Workers Exposed to Pesticides: Evaluation with the Comet and Buccal Micronucleus Cytome Assays." *Mutation Research* 752, nos. 1–2 (April 2013): 28–33.

Black, M. H., R. M. Watanabe, E. Trigo, et al. "High-Fat Diet Associated with Obesity-Medicated Insulin Resistance and β-cell Dysfunction in Mexican Americans." *Journal of Nutrition* 143, no. 4 (April 2013): 479–85.

Bashan N., Bluher, M., I. Shai, et al. "Activated Ask1-MKK4-p38MAPK/JNK Stress Signaling Pathway in Human Omental Fat Tissue May Link Macrophage Infiltration to Whole-Body Insulin Sensitivity." *Journal of Clinical Endocrinology & Metabolism* 94, no. 7 (2009): 2507.

Brattabakk, H. R., I. Arbo, S. Aagaard, et al. *OMICS* 17, no. 1 (January 2013): 41–52.

Cardozo, L. F., L. M. Pedruzzi, P. Stenvinkel, et al. "Nutritional Strategies to Modulate Inflammation and Oxidative Stress Pathways via Activation of the Master Antioxidant Switch Nrf2." *Biochimie* 95, no. 8 (2013): 1525–33.

Centers for Disease Control and Prevention. "ADHD Data and Statistics." http://www.cdc.gov/ncbddd/adhd/data.html (accessed November 2, 2014).

Centers for Disease Control and Prevention. "An Estimated 1 in 10 U.S. Adults Report Depression." http://www.cdc.gov/features/dsdepression/ (accessed November 2, 2014).

Collins, A., A. Asqueta, and S. Langie. "Effects of Micronutrients on DNA Repair." *European Journal of Nutrition* 51 (February 2012): 261–79.

Getek, M., N. Czech, K. Fizia, et al. "Nutrigenomics—Bioactive Dietary Components." *Postępy Higieny i Medycyny Doświadczalnej* 67 (April 2013): 255–60.

Hamilton, L. D., and C. M. Meston. "Chronic Stress and Sexual Function in Women." *Journal of Sexual Medicine* 10, no. 10 (October 2013): 2443–54.

Jiménez-Chillaŕon, J. C., R. Diaz, D. Martinez, et al. "The Role of Nutrition on Epigenetic Modifications and Their Implications on Health." *Biochimie* 94, no. 11 (November 2012): 2242–63.

Kesari, K. K., M. H. Siddiqui, R. Meena, et al. "Cell Phone Radiation Exposure on Brain and Associated Biological Systems." *Indian Journal of Experimental Biology* 51, no. 3 (March 2013): 187–200.

Khayat, C. B., E. O. Costa, M. W. Goncalves, et al. "Assessment of DNA Damage in Brazilian Workers Occupationally Exposed to Pesticides: A Study from Central Brazil." *Environmental Science and Pollution Research International* 20, no. 10 (October 2013): 7334–40.

Kropat, C., D. Mueller, U. Boettler, et al. "Modulation of Nrf2-Dependent Gene Transcription by Bilberry Anthocyanins in Vivo." *Molecular Nutrition and Food Research* 57, no. 3 (2013): 545–50.

Lee, M. S., K. A. Kim, and H. S. Kim. "Role of Pancreatic β-Cell Death and Cell Death-Associated Inflammation in Diabetes." *Current Molecular Medicine* 12, no. 10 (December 2012): 1297–1310.

Leone, A., and L. Landini. "Vascular Pathology from Smoking: Look at the Microcirculation!" *Current Vascular Pharmacology* 11, no. 4 (July 2013): 524–530.

Lopez-Armada, M., R. Riveiro-Naveira, C. Vaamonde-Garcia, et al. "Mitochondrial Dysfunction and the Inflammatory Response." *Mitochondrion* 13 (2013): 106–18.

Lu, Y., B .Huang, and Y. Huang. "Reactive Oxygen Species Formation and Apoptosis in Human Peripheral Blood Mononuclear Cell Induced by 900 MHz Phone Radiation." *Oxidative Medicine and Cellular Longevity* (2012): 740280.

Merz, Beverly. "Cell Membrane Defects in Mental Illness." *Journal of the American Medical Association* 248, no. 6 (1982): 633.

Moon, M., M. Kim, I. Jung, et al. "Bisphenol A Impairs Mitochondrial Function in the Liver at Doses Below the No Observed Adverse Effect Level." *Journal of Korean Medical Science* 27, no. 6 (June 2012): 644–52.

Muris. D. M., A. J. Houben, M. T. Schram, et al. "Microvascular Dysfunction: An Emerging Pathway in the Pathogenesis of Obesity-Related Insulin Resistance." *Reviews in Endocrine Metabolic Disorders* 14, no. 1 (March 2013): 29–38.

Nagai, M., Y. Morikawa, K. Kitaoka, et al. "Effects of Fatigue on Immune Function in Nurses Performing Shift Work." *Journal of Occupational Health* 53, no. 5 (2011): 312–19.

Narayan, K. M. V., J. P. Boyle, T. J. Thompson, et al. "Lifetime Risk for Diabetes Mellitus in the United States." *Journal of the American Medical Association* 290, no. 14 (October 2003): 1884–90.

O'Donovan, A., A. Tomiyama, J. Lin, et al. *Brain Behavior and Immunology* 26, no. 4 (May 2012): 573–79.

Puca, A., A. Carrizzo, F. Villa, et al. "Vascular Ageing: The Role of Oxidative Stress." *International Journal of Biochemistry & Cell Biology* 45 (2013): 556–59.

Rayssiquier, Y., E. Gueux, W. Nowacki, et al. "High Fructose Consumption Combined with Low Dietary Magnesium Intake May Increase the Incidence of the Metabolic Syndrome by Inducing Inflammation." *Magnesium Research* 19, no. 4 (December 2006): 237–43.

Sanacora, G., and M. Banasr. "From Pathophysiology to Novel Antidepressant Drugs: Glial Contributions to the Pathology and Treatment of Mood Disorders." *Biological Psychiatry* 73, no. 12 (June 2013): 1172–79.

Trayhurn, P. "Hypoxia and Adipose Tissue Function and Dysfunction in Obesity." *Physiological Reviews* 93, no. 1 (January 2013): 1–21.

Van Sloten, T. T., M. T. Schram, M. C. Adriaanse, et al. "Endothelial Dysfunction Is Associated with a Greater Depressive Symptom Score in a General Elderly Population: The Hoorn Study." *Psychological Medicine* 44, no. 7 (August 2013): 1–14.

Weischer, M., S. Bojesen, R. Cawthon, et al. "Atherosclerosis: Short Telomere Length, Myocardial Infarction, Ischemic Heart Disease, and Early Death." *Arterior Sclerosis, Thrombosis, and Vascular Biology* 32, no. 3 (March 2012): 822–29.

Wilkins, J. T., H. Ning, J. Berry, et al. "Lifetime Risk and Years Lived Free of Total Cardiovascular Disease." *Journal of the American Medical Association* 308, no. 17 (November 2012): 1795–1801.

Wolf, A., B. Bauer, and A. M. Hartz. "ABC Transporters and the Alzheimer's Disease Enigma." *Front Psychiatry* 3 (June 2012): 54.

CHAPTER 2

Allen, L. A. Jr. "Adrenal Fatigue." *International Journal of Pharmaceutical Compounding* 17, no. 1 (January–February 2013): 39–44.

Arner, P., S. Bernard, M. Salepour, et al. "Dynamics of Human Adipose Lipid Turnover in Health and Metabolic Disease." *Nature* 478, no. 7367 (September 2011): 110–13.

Cocchi, M., L. Tonello, F. Gabrielli, et al. "Depression, Osteoporosis, Serotonin and Cell Membrane Viscosity between Biology and Philosophical Anthropology." *Annals of General Psychiatry* 10 (2011): 9.

Head, K., and G. Kelly, "Nutrients and Botanicals for Treatment of Stress: Adrenal Fatigue, Neurotransmitter Imbalance, Anxiety, and Restless Sleep." *Alternative Medicine Review* 14 (2009): 114–40.

Lang, C. H., X. Liu, G. Nystrom, et al. "Acute Effects of Growth Hormne in Alcohol-fed Rats." *Alcohol and Alcoholism* 35, no. 2 (March–April 2000): 148–58.

Miller, Andrew. "Depression and Immunity: A Role for T cells?" *Brain, Behavior, and Immunity* 24, no. 1 (January 2010): 1–8.

Nutt, D. J. "Relationship of Neurotransmitters to the Symptoms of Major Depressive Disorder." *Journal of Clinical Psychiatry* 69, Supplement E1 (2008): 4–7.

Palazzo, L. S., M. Carlotto, and D. Aerts. "Burnout Syndrome: Population-Based Study on Public Servants." *Revisa Saúde Pública* 46, no. 6 (December 2012): 1066–73.

Patrick, Lyn. "Thyroid Disruption: Mechanisms and Clinical Implications in Human Health." *Alternative Medicine Review* 14 (2009): 326–46.

Pepin, E., and M.-L. Peyot. "β-Cell Failure in Diet-Induced Obese Mice Stratified According to Body Weight Gain: Secretory Dysfunction and Altered Islet Lipid

Metabolism without Steatosis or Reduced β-Cell Mass." *Diabetes* 59, no. 9 (September 2010): 2178–87.

Pranjic, N., S. Nuhbegovic, S. Brekalo-Lazarevic, et al. "Is Adrenal Exhaustion Synonym of Syndrome Burnout at Workplace?" *Collegium Antropologicum* 36, no. 3 (September 2012): 911–19.

CHAPTER 3

Alhola, P., and P. Polo-Kantola. "Sleep Deprivation: Impact on Cognitive Performance." *Neuropsychiatric Disorders Treatment* 3, no. 5 (October 2007): 553–67.

Blask, David. "Melatonin, Sleep Disturbance and Cancer Risk." *Sleep Medicine Reviews* 13 (2009): 257–64.

Ford, D. E., and D. B. Kamerow. "Epidemiologic Study of Sleep Disturbances and Psychiatric Disorders. An Opportunity for Prevention?" *Journal of the American Medical Association* 262, no. 11 (September 1989): 1479–84.

Killgore, W. D. "Effects of Sleep Deprivation on Cognition." *Progressive Brain Research* 185 (2010): 105–29.

Knutson, K., K. Spiegal, and E. Van Cauter. "The Metabolic Consequences of Sleep Deprivation." *Sleep Medicine Review* 11, no. 3 (June 2007): 163–78.

McNamara, P., S. Auerbach, P. Johnson, et al. "Impact of REM Sleep on Distortions of Self-Concept, Mood and Memory in Depressed/Anxious Participants." *Journal of Affective Disorders* 122, no. 3 (May 2010): 198–207.

National Alliance on Mental Illness. "The Impact and Cost of Mental Illness: The Case of Depression." http://www.nami.org/Template.cfm?Section=Policymakers_ Toolkit&Template=/ContentManagement/ContentDisplay.cfm&ContentID=19043 (accessed November 2, 2014)

Piletz, J. E., A. Halaris, O. Iqbal, et al. "Pro-Inflammatory Biomarkers in Depression: Treatment with Venlafaxine." *World Journal of Biological Psychiatry* 10, no. 4 (2009): 313–23.

Rosales-Legarde, A., J. Armony, and M. Corsi-Cabrera. "Enhanced Emotional Reactivity after Selective REM Sleep Deprivation in Humans: An fMRI Study." *Frontiers in Behavioral Neuroscience* 6 (2012): 25.

University Hospitals Case Medical Centre. "Lack of Sleep Found to Be a New Risk Factor for Aggressive Breast Cancers." *Science Daily* (August 27, 2012). http://www.sciencedaily.com/releases/2012/08/120827113359.htm (accessed November 2, 2014).

University Hospitals Case Medical Centre. "Lack of Sleep Found to Be a New Risk Factor for Colon Cancer." *Science Daily* (February 8, 2011). http://www.sciencedaily.com/releases/2011/02/110208112741.htm (accessed November 2, 2014).

Van Caute, E., K. Spiegel, E. Tasali, et al. "Metabolic Consequences of Sleep and Sleep Loss." *Sleep Medicine* 9, Supplement 1 (September 2008): S23–A28.

Winokur, A., K. A. Gary, S. Rodner, et al. "Depression, Sleep Physiology, and Antidepressant Drugs." *Depression and Anxiety* 14, no. 1 (2001): 19–28.

Zhao, G., E. S. Ford, S. Dhingra, et al. "Depression and Anxiety among US Adults: Associations with Body Mass Index." *International Journal of Obesity (London)* 33, no. 22 (February 2009): 257–66.

CHAPTER 4

Asthma and Allergy Foundation of America. "Food Allergies." https://www.aafa.org/display.cfm?id=9&sub=20&cont=286 (accessed November 2, 2014).

Collin, A. R., A. Azqueta, and S. A. Langie. "Effects of Micronutrients on DNA Repair." *European Journal of Nutrition* 51, no. 3 (April 2012): 261–79.

Depeint, F., W. R. Bruce, N. Shangari, et al. "Mitochondrial Function and Toxicity: Role of B Vitamins on the One-Carbon Transfer Pathways." *Chemico-Biological Interactions* 163, nos. 1–2 (October 2006): 113–32.

Food Allergy Research & Education. "*Facts and Statistics.*" http://www.foodallergy.org/facts-and-stats (accessed November 2, 2014).

Hellmann, Hanjo. "Vitamin B_6: A Molecule for Human Health?" *Molecules* 15 (2010): 442–59.

Kidd, Parris. "Neurodegeneration from Mitochondrial Insufficiency: Nutrients, Stem Cells, Growth Factors, and Prospects for Brain Rebuilding Using Integrative Management." *Alternative Medicine Review* 10 (2005): 268–93.

Koopula, S., H. Kumar, S. More, et al. "Recent Updates in Redox Regulation and Free Radical Scavenging Effects by Herbal Products in Experimental Models of Parkinson's Disease." *Molecules* 17 (2012): 11391–420.

National Institute of Diabetes and Digestive and Kidney Diseases. "Celiac Disease." http://digestive.niddk.nih.gov/ddiseases/pubs/celiac/ (accessed May 4, 2014).

Nicholson, G. L. "Mitochondrial Dysfunction and Chronic Disease: Treatment with Natural Supplements." *Alternative Therapies in Health and Medicine* 20, Supplement 1 (Winter 2014): 18–25.

Poljsak, B. "Strategies for Reducing or Preventing the Generation of Oxidative Stress." *Oxidative Medicine and Cell Longevity* (2011): 194586.

Virmani, A., L. Pinto, Z. Binienda, et al. "Food, Nutrigenomics, and Neurodegeneration-Neuroprotection by What You Eat!" *Molecular Neurobiology* 48, no. 2 (October 2013): 353–62.

Wall, S., J. Oh, A. Diers, et al. "Oxidative Modification of Proteins: An Emerging Mechanism of Cell Signaling." *Frontiers in Physiology* 3 (September 2012): 1–9.

CHAPTER 5

Anxiety and Depression Association of America. "Exercise for Stress and Anxiety." (2011). http://www.adaa.org/living-with-anxiety/managing-anxiety/exercise-stress-and-anxiety (accessed November 2, 2014).

Baar, K. "Training for Endurance and Strength: Lessons from Cell Signaling." *Medicine & Science in Sports & Exercise* 38, no. 11 (November 2006): 1939–44.

Centers for Disease Control and Prevention. "Why Strength Training?" http://www.cdc.gov/physicalactivity/growingstronger/why/ (accessed November 2, 2014).

Deslandes, Andrea. "The Biological Clock Keeps Ticking, But Exercise May Turn It Back." *Arquivos de Neuro-Siquiatry* 71, no. 2 (February 2013): 113–18.

Frederickson, B., M. Cohn, K. Coffey, et al. "Open Hearts Build Lives: Positive Emotions, Induced through Loving-Kindness Meditation, Build Consequential Personal Resources." *Journal of Personality and Social Psychology* 95, no. 5 (November 2008): 1045–62.

Hanssen, K. E., N. H. Kyamme, T. S. Nilsen, et al. "The Effect of Strength Training Volume on Satellite Cells, Myogenic Regulatory Factors, and Growth Factors." *Scandinavian Journal of Medicine and Science in Sports* 23, no. 6 (December 2013): 728–39.

Khorvash, M., A. Askari, F. Rafiemanzelat, et al. "An Investigation on the Effect of Strength and Endurance Training on Depression, Anxiety and C-Reactive Protein's Inflammatory Biomarker Changes." *Journal of Research in Medicine and Science* 17, no. 11 (November 2012): 1072–76.

Ludlow, A. T., J. B. Zimmerman, S. Witkowski, et al. "Relationship between Physical Activity Level, Telomere Length, and Telomerase Activity." *Medicine & Science in Sports & Exercise* 40, no. 10 (October 2008): 1764–71.

Martin Ginis, K. A., J. J. Eng, K. P. Arbour, et al. "Mind over Muscle? Sex Differences in the Relationship between Body Image Change and Subjective and Objective Physical Changes Following a 12-Week Strength-Training Program." *Body Image* 2, no. 4 (December 2005): 363–72.

Reidy, P. T., D. K. Walker, J. M. Dickinson, et al. "Protein Blend Ingestion Following Resistance Exercise Promotes Human Muscle Protein Synthesis." *Journal of Nutrition* 143, no. 4 (April 2013): 410–16.

Schuenke, M. D., R. P. Mikat, and J. M. McBride. "Effect of an Acute Period of Resistance Exercise on Excess Post-Exercise Oxygen Consumption: Implications for Body Mass Management." *European Journal of Applied Physiology* 86 (2002): 411–17.

Thomas, G. A., W. J. Kraemer, B. A. Comstock, et al. "Effects of Resistance Exercise and Obesity Level on Ghrelin and Cortisol in Men." *Metabolism* 61, no. 6 (June 2012): 860–68.

Thomas, G. A., W. J. Kraemer, M. J. Kennett, et al. "Immunoreactive and Bioactive Growth Hormone Responses to Resistance Exercise in Men Who Are Lean or Obese." *Journal of Applied Physiology* 111, no. 2 (August 2011): 265–72.

Trapp, E. G., D. J. Chisholm, J. Freund, et al. "The Effects of High-Intensity Intermittent Exercise Training on Fat Loss and Fasting Insulin Levels of Young Women." *International Journal of Obesity* 32 (2008): 684–91.

CHAPTER 6

Axelsson, J., T. Sundelin, M. Ingre, et al. "Beauty Sleep: Experimental Study on the Perceived Health and Attractiveness of Sleep Deprived People." *British Medical Journal* 341 (2010): 6614.

Bruusgaard, J. C., I. B. Johansen, I. M. Egner, et al. "Myonuclei Acquired by Overload Exercise Precede Hypertrophy and Are Not Lost on Detraining." *Proceedings of the National Academy of Science of the USA* 107, no. 34 (August 24, 2010): 15111–16.

Chaput, Jean-Phillippe. "Short Sleep Duration Promoting Overconsumption of Food: A Reward-Driving Eating Behavior?" *Sleep* 33, no. 9 (September 1, 2010): 1135–36.

Comai, S., and G. Gobbi. "Unveiling the Role of Melatonin Mt2 Receptors in Sleep, Anxiety and Other Neuropsychiatric Diseases: A Novel Target in Psychopharmacology." *Journal of Psychiatry and Neuroscience* 39, no. 1 (January 2014): 6–21.

Currie, T. E., and A. C. Little. "The Relative Importance of the Face and Body in Judgments of Human Physical Attractiveness." *Evolution and Human Behavior* (2009). doi: 10.1016/j.evolhumbehav.2009.06.005.

Gujar, N., S. A. McDonald, M. Nishida, et al. "A Role for REM Sleep in Recalibrating the Sensitivity of the Human Brain to Specific Emotions." *Cerebral Cortex* 21 (January 2011): 115–23.

Kostoglou-Athanassiou, Ifigenia. "Therapeutic Applications of Melatonin." *Therapies and Advances in Endocrinal Metabolism* 41, no. 1 (2013): 13–24.

Lemola, S., T. Ledermann, and E. M. Friedman. "Variability of Sleep Duration Is Related to Subjective Sleep Quality and Subjective Well-Being: An Acitgraphy Study." *PLOS One* 8, no. 8 (August 14, 2013): e71292.

Myllymäki, T., H. Kyröläinen, K. Savolainen, et al. *Journal of Sleep Research* 20, no. 1, pt. 2 (March 2011): 146–53.

Nunes, A., and M. Sousa. "Use of Valerian in Anxiety and Sleep Disorders: What Is the Best Evidence?" *Acta Medica Portugesa* 24, Supplement 4 (December 2011): 961–66.

Van der Helm, E., and M. P. Walker. "Overnight Therapy? The Role of Sleep in Emotional Brain Processing." *Psychological Bulletin* 135, no. 5 (September 2009): 731–48.

INDEX